WEIGHT TRAINING
for Life

Fifth Edition

James L. Hesson
Black Hills State University

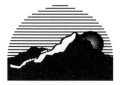

Morton Publishing Company
925 W. Kenyon, Unit 12
Englewood, Colorado 80110
http://www.morton-pub.com

Dedication

To the wind beneath my wings, the creator of all that is, the source of my inspiration and strength, the source of my knowledge and wisdom, the great spirit that is within all of us, and the great spirit through which we are all joined as one in the endless cycle of life.

To Margie, Jennifer, and David, for their love and support.

To all of the teachers, coaches, friends, and colleagues who have shared their time, energy, and knowledge with me.

To all of my students who have taught me, and who continue to teach me, how to help them learn.

To my parents, Jack and Gladys Hesson, who taught me the basic values and attitudes that have made all other learning and accomplishment possible.

Printed in the United States of America

10 9 8 7 6 5 4 3 2 1

ISBN: 0-89582-523-6

Preface

Student

Weight Training for Life has been written to you and for you. Learning about weight training by the trial-and-error method can be difficult, embarrassing, and confusing. We hope this book will make learning simple, painless, easy, and fun. Its purpose is to help you build a good foundation of current knowledge and practice in beginning weight training. All of the exercise information in this book is consistent with the recommendations of the National Strength and Conditioning Association (NSCA) and the American College of Sports Medicine (ACSM). This book does not attempt to include everything to be known about weight training.

This is a book for beginners, not for exercise physiologists or advanced-strength athletes. Most of all, this is a book to help you get started *weight training for life*.

Teacher

Weight Training for Life has been written to help you and to help your students. It does not attempt to cover everything you know about weight training, but it does attempt to organize some basic information for you and your students.

One common challenge for most weight training teachers is time. Answer the following questions quickly.

- Do you have enough class time to tell your students all that you wish you could about weight training?
- Are your students always present, on time, and alert for your weight training lectures?
- Do you have other classes to prepare for?
- Are you paid for talking or for ensuring that learning takes place?
- Do you ever get bored presenting the same beginning weight training information year after year and class after class?
- Have you ever forgotten to mention some basic information you wanted your students to know?
- Could you be more productive if you did not have to repeat the same basic information again and again?
- Would your students learn more effectively if they were required to actively seek information?
- Do you have enough class time to present all the information you want and still have enough exercise time?
- Do you teach more than one weight training class?
- Have you ever noticed how the right tool can help you complete a task easier, faster, and better?

This book is a tool that can help you perform your task of teaching weight training. It can make your performance of this task better and, at the same time, easier. A book will never replace you as a teacher because your role is much more important, dynamic, and complex. Your responsibility is to create a stimulating learning environment, to motivate, to provide direction, and to give feedback.

The material in this book can be covered in any order you choose. You also are encouraged to add or delete any material you wish. Based on the feedback I have received, there seems to be an infinite variety of ways to help beginners learn about weight training.

This tool can be more effective if we work together. As you use the book, let me know how we can improve it to help you and your students. To those of you who used the first four editions and sent your suggestions for improvements, you will find most of these in this fifth edition. Thank you for making this revision possible and for making it better.

JLH

Acknowledgments

I would like to thank everyone who helped make this fifth edition possible. Special appreciation is given to the following individuals.

Margie Hesson for serving as a contributing author of this book. Her professional and personal knowledge of exercise and healthy lifestyles brought valuable changes to this new edition. Margie's careful proof reading of the manuscript, in addition to her writing contributions, brought the female perspective to the presentation of the material making this a more balanced text for men and women.

Dr. Larry Tentinger for serving as a contributing author.

All of the **Weight Training Teachers** who answered our questions and helped to shape this new edition.

Jon Kelley of **Jon's Photography** in Colorado Springs for his excellent photography.

Eric Risberg for his professional photography.

Doug Duran and **Erik Berger** for their expert advice and help during the most recent photo session.

Andre Morrow for all he did to arrange the previous photo session and to make this book possible. Andre, you are the greatest.

Leslie Araya, Courtney Bennigson, Erik Berger, Sara Brinkley, Grant Conklin, Jason Gatson, Brett McClure, Anna Lissa I. Nool, Chris Parker, and **Jason Yeske** for their time energy, ideas, encouragement, and patience as models.

Jeff Boyle for allowing us to take new photographs in Gold's Gym of Colorado Springs.

Werner and **Sharon Hoeger** for being generous and caring to share their knowledge and material with us so we can share it with you.

Nautilus and **Universal Gym Equipment, Inc.** for the excellent photographs.

David Hesson for his help in selecting photographs.

Kristi Willenberg for her help with internet sites and proof reading.

Jim Bryant for his friendship and helpful attitude as well as everything he did for me to make the earlier editions of this book possible.

Milton Wilder for his support, encouragement, and friendship. As you know Milton, this book never would have happened without you. Thank you.

Tom Kidd for his early encouragement and support of an extremely thin and weak young boy. He supported my early weight training at a time when weight training was not popular and was not recommended by most coaches. It took a lot of courage to stand up for what you believed to be right, when all of the other coaches thought you were wrong. Scientific research has since proven that you were right and they were wrong.

Jake Geier for teaching me the difference between "producers" and "excusers."

Phil Allsen for his friendship as well as his continuing faith in me and support of my professional and personal development.

Joanne Saliger for making this such an attractive and functional book.

Ruth Horton for helping me complete five editions of this book.

Doug Morton for being an outstanding person, and friend, as well as an excellent publisher.

Contents

1 **What, Who, and Why** **1**

What is Weight Training?   1
Who Trains with Weights?   1
Who Should Participate in Weight Training?   2
Why Weight Training?   4
Participate in Your Own Creation   6

2 **Questions, Concerns, and Answers** **7**

3 **Muscle Structure and Function** **11**

Your Muscular System   11
Characteristics of Muscle Tissue   11
Types of Muscle Tissue   11
The Musculoskeletal System as a Lever System   12
The Structure of Skeletal Muscle   12
Muscle Contraction and Exercise Movements   13
Motor Unit   14
Muscle Atrophy and Hypertrophy   15

4 **Warm-Up, Flexibility, and Stretching** **17**

Warm-Up   17
Flexibility   17
Stretching   18
Joints to Stretch   19
When to Stretch   19

5 **Safe and Effective Weight Training** . . **21**

Medical Clearance   21
Clothing   21
Performing a Weight Training Exercise   22
Additional Considerations for Machine Exercises   24
Training Partner   26
Spotting   26
Safety   28

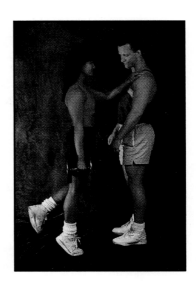

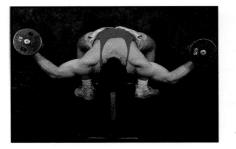

6 🍃 **A Beginning Weight Training Program . . 29**

Free Weights and Machines   29
Grips   29
Basic Lifts   31
Beginning Exercises   32
Frequency and Resistance   33
The First Six Weeks   33
Guidelines for Productive Training   34

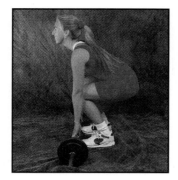

Introduction to Exercises   39

Division of Exercises   39
Major Muscles of the Human Body   40

7 🍃 **Chest Exercises** **41**

Chest   42
Chest/Back   48

8 🍃 **Back Exercises** **51**

Back (Lats)   52
Upper Back (Traps)   58

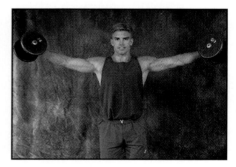

9 🍃 **Shoulder Exercises** **59**

10 🍃 **Arm Exercises** **69**

Upper Arm (Elbow Flexion)   70
Upper Arm (Elbow Extension)   74
Forearm   80

11 🍃 **Leg Exercises** **83**

Hip and Knee Extension   84
Hip Extension   90
Hip Flexion   91
Knee Extension   92
Knee Flexion   93
Ankle Plantar Flexion   94

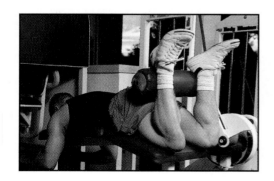

12 Abdominal and Back Extension Exercises. **99**

Trunk Flexion (Abdominals) 100
Trunk and Hip Flexion (Abdominals and Hip Flexors) 102
Trunk Extension (Erector Spinae) 106

13 Nutrition, Rest, and Drugs **109**

Nutrition 109
The "Secret" Weight training Diet 114
Nutrient Supplementation 116
Weight Gain 116
Weight Loss 116
Rest 117
Drugs 118

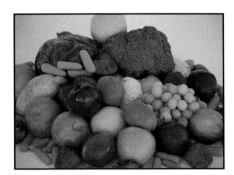

14 Record-Keeping and Progress **125**

Record Keeping 125
Measuring Progress 127
Evaluating Progress 129

15 A Formula For Success. **137**

What is Success? 137
A Formula for Success 137
Writing Weight Training Goals 139

16 Planning a Weight Training Program. **143**

Basic Weight Training Principles 143
Considerations in Planning Your Weight Training Program 143
Suggested Lifetime Fitness Weight Training Programs 146

17 Advanced Weight Training **153**

Progressive Overload 153
Increasing Exercise Intensity 153
Total Body and Spilt Routines 154
Fixed Systems 154
Variable Systems 155
Training Equipment 156

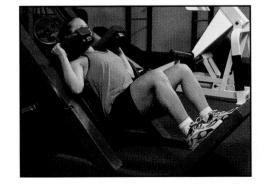

18 ◖ Tips for Sticking With It 157

Motivation   157
Enjoyment   157
Importance   157
Priority   157
Time   157
Record   158
Reward   158
Learn   158
Social   158
Support   158
Identity   158
Place   158
Convenience   158
Instruction   158
Variety   158
Fitness   159
Success   159
Appearance   159
Image   159
Regularity   159
Habit   159
Simple Home Training for Busy People   159
Weight Training for Life   160

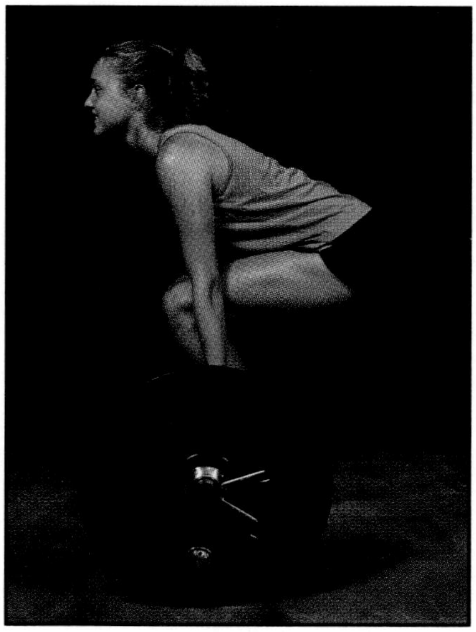

Appendix A ◖ Internet Sites 163

References and Suggested Readings 165

Index 167

What, Who, and Why

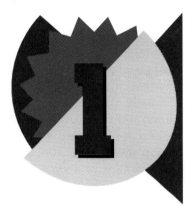

WHAT IS WEIGHT TRAINING?

Weight training is a form of resistance exercise. Weights of different sizes can be added to, or taken from, the total load to arrive at the correct resistance for each exercise and each muscle group.

Weight training exercises are done for different reasons. The following categories of weight trainers may help you understand why so many different kinds of weight training programs exist.

WHO TRAINS WITH WEIGHTS?

Olympic Lifters

Olympic-style weight lifting is a competitive sport. The objective in olympic-style lifting is to see who can lift the most total weight overhead using two different lifts. The two olympic-style lifts are the snatch and the clean-and-jerk.

The *snatch lift* requires that the weight be lifted in one continuous movement from the floor to a position in which the weight is overhead and both arms are straight. The lifter may drop below the weight to catch it overhead but must rise to a stationary standing position to complete the lift.

In the *clean-and-jerk lift* the weight must first be brought from the floor to a position on the upper chest and shoulders. Then, from a standing position the weight is thrust overhead to a straight-arm finish.

The winner is the individual with the highest total when the snatch and the clean-and-jerk lifts are added together. The competitors are grouped into different body weight classifications so they are competing against others who are approximately the same size.

Power Lifters

Power lifters compete in three lifts: the *bench press*, the *squat*, and the *dead lift*. The winner is the lifter with the highest total for the three lifts. These competitors also are grouped by body weight so they are competing against other lifters who are approximately the same size.

Body Builders

Body builders participate in competition that is more art than sport. Through weight training they create a living sculpture using the human body as the clay. Body builders attempt to develop maximum muscular size while maintaining a balanced appearance (symmetry) and a high degree of muscular visibility (definition). In this competition the appearance of the body is most important.

Athletes

Since the rehabilitation work of Dr. Thomas De-Lorme following World War II, progressive resistance exercise has gradually gained acceptance by the medical profession and the coaching profession. A dramatic change has taken place during the last 50 years. In the 1950s and early 1960s most coaches told their athletes that they should not lift weights. During the 1970s lifting became more acceptable for athletes. In the 1980s and 1990s most coaches required their athletes to lift weights.

Most top-level athletes now use some form of weight training to improve their sports performance and to recover from sports injuries. Because skeletal muscles are responsible for all voluntary human movement, athletes who increase the functional ability of their muscular system almost always improve their sports performance.

Recently, there has been an increased focus on the opposing muscle groups. In the early years of weight training to improve athletic performance, much of the emphasis was placed on the muscles that produce the successful sports movements. Although it did strengthen the desired muscles, and performance did improve, this type of training often created an imbalance of strength surrounding a joint. Occasionally the stronger muscles on one side of the joint overpowered and injured the weaker muscles on the other side of the joint.

Good weight training programs for athletes now include exercises for balanced development to increase performance and reduce the risk of injury.

Patients

Physicians and physical therapists frequently prescribe progressive resistance exercise as a part of the rehabilitation program for people who have been injured. By training with weights, these patients regain strength, muscle size, and functional ability after an injury.

Physical Fitness Enthusiasts

Many people who exercise for health and physical fitness are discovering the benefits of weight training. Most of the people in this category want to look better, feel better, and be healthier.

Weight training and the increase of muscle tissue should be an important part of any fat loss program. Many have overlooked the benefits of weight training for fat loss because of the focus on calories spent during an exercise session. As many as 75 calories per day may be used to support the energy needs of one pound of muscle tissue. As few as 3 calories per day may be used to support the energy needs of one pound of fat tissue. Because muscle is active tissue that consumes calories, and fat is inactive tissue that stores calories, those who

are trying to lose body fat should increase their muscle mass.

Weight Trainers

Anyone who trains with weights may be considered a weight trainer. This book has been written primarily for those who are just beginning to lift weights, and for the physical fitness enthusiast, with the hope that if they get off to a good start, they will participate in *weight training for life*.

WHO SHOULD PARTICIPATE IN WEIGHT TRAINING?

Everyone who has a muscular system can benefit from a regular program of progressive resistance exercise. Therefore, almost everyone should participate in *weight training for life*.

Men and Women

Some of the benefits of weight training for men and women include more strength, increased muscle size, greater muscle endurance, improved appearance, higher self-esteem, and better sports performance. The location and function of the skeletal muscles is the same in men and women. Research during the last three decades has indicated that the weight training principles, methods, programs, and exercises that have worked well for men work equally well for women. Weight training exercises are the same for men and women. Although there are no "men's exercises" or "women's exercises" men and women may choose to develop different muscle groups which may affect their selection of exercises.

Is weight training an appropriate activity for girls and women? Absolutely! All women achieve increases in muscular strength when they participate in properly planned weight training programs. Most women do not experience as much increase in muscle size as most men on the same training program. This seems to be related to lower levels of the hormone testosterone and a lower number of muscle fibers, particularly in the upper body.

Weight training will not make a woman appear masculine or cause a woman to develop any secondary male characteristics such as a deeper voice, facial hair, or thicker body hair. These secondary gender characteristics are caused primarily by hormones. During puberty boys begin producing higher levels of male hormones which produce the secondary sex characteristics we associate with males. At puberty girls begin producing higher levels of female hormones which produce secondary sex characteristics we associate with females. This hormone production is extremely variable from one person to another. As a result of a well-planned weight training program, both men and women tend to develop a strong, firm, healthy, attractive appearance.

Children

Children can gain important benefits through a carefully planned and closely supervised weight training program. Those who participate in weight training can gain strength, improve their self-image, increase their level of physical fitness, improve their sports performance, and possibly reduce their risk of youth sport injury.

The risk of injury from weight training during participation in a carefully planned and closely supervised weight training program for children is low. The few injuries that have been reported usually have occurred during improperly performed overhead lifts. Too much weight, improper technique, poorly planned programs, and a lack of supervision have been contributing factors.

Those who are responsible for planning and supervising weight training programs for children must be trained and qualified in this area. Each exercise, along with the spotting techniques for that exercise, must be taught and demonstrated correctly. The young weight trainer should not be allowed to train alone without proper supervision and a trained spotter. The training area should be clean, bright, attractive, and large enough to perform each lift safely.

Training programs for children should focus on all-around physical development, not just strength training. Strength is only one aspect of physical development.

Children should train with moderate to light weights that can be handled for fairly high repetitions. The National Strength and Conditioning Association recommends 6 to 15 repetitions in each set. This means that a child should not be allowed to lift a weight unless he or she can complete at least 6 correct repetitions with that weight. Children should not attempt 1-repetition maximum lifts.

Children should be allowed to participate in weight training voluntarily. If young children are forced to participate in weight training they are more likely to develop a negative attitude toward this beneficial activity. If they develop a negative attitude, they probably will not participate in *weight training for life.*

After puberty and during adolescence, as hormone changes occur, children begin to experience greater physical changes as a result of a weight training program. During this time strict exercise form should be maintained, and close qualified adult supervision is critical. Boys at this age seem to have an overwhelming urge to find out who can lift the most weight one time. Of course, what they often find out is how much they cannot lift one time. The risk of injury is too high.

As young people near full growth and full physical maturity, weight training can have its most dramatic positive effects on physical performance, appearance, and self-confidence. This is a time when they can handle heavier exercise loads and more intense exercise programs. To maximize safety and progress, however, the emphasis must always remain on correct exercise technique. Many young men resort to poor exercise technique to move a heavier weight. This can result in injury. Weight training exercises performed correctly rarely result in injury.

Adults

During the aging process, strength and muscle mass decline. How much of this decrease is a result of biological aging and how much is a result of a sedentary lifestyle? Very little of the decline in strength during the adult years is a result of natural aging. Individuals living in societies that are advanced in technology and automation reveal a much greater loss of strength and mobility with aging. This may result from inactivity and a failure to maintain the muscular system.

Many individuals in the wage-earning adult years think they do not have time for weight training, when weight training actually is an efficient form of exercise. With weight training, a muscle group can be isolated and worked very hard in an extremely short time. A stimulus strong enough to maintain strength, or to cause a gain in the strength of a muscle group, may be achieved in about one minute with some weight training programs. This is a greater strength gain stimulus than the same muscle group would achieve in hours of participating in most adult recreational activities.

All of the major muscles in the body can be exercised in 15 to 20 minutes. If this weight training program is performed two or three times each week, that is an investment of 30 to 60 minutes a week. Each week has 168 hours, and you can maintain your strength during your adult years by investing approximately 1 hour per week in weight training. If your time for exercise is limited, weight training is one of the fastest ways to maintain or increase the functioning of your muscular system. It is important for adults to continue *weight training for life*.

Older Adults

At what age should adults stop weight training? Never! Humans should not use age as an excuse to stop weight training. Some older adults may be advised by their physicians to stop weight training because of medical problems, but as long as there is no medical reason to quit, there is no reason to stop weight training at any certain age. Weight training programs, however, do have to be modified with age.

Sometime in their 60s, 70s, 80s, or 90s, most older adults experience a more rapid decline in physical performance. It has been difficult to determine how much of this decline is a result of the decrease in physical activity that often accompanies retirement and how much relates to a person's decision that it is time to get old and to act old. In either case, older adults must maintain their muscular system if they wish to retain their freedom and their mobility. Therefore, older adults should participate in *weight training for life*.

Everyone

Weight training is an efficient form of exercise to develop and maintain your muscular system. Though your goals and training programs will change as you progress through life, weight training is a valuable lifetime activity that you should continue. Everyone should participate in some form of *weight training for life*.

WHY WEIGHT TRAINING?

Surgeon General's Report

The Centers for Disease Control and Prevention (CDC) released *Physical Activity and Health: A Report of the Surgeon General*. One of the findings reported was that "Approximately 15 percent of U.S. adults engage regularly (3 times a week for at least 20 minutes) in vigorous physical activity during leisure time." Which, of course, means that 85% do not. One of the major conclusions in the report was that "people of all ages, both male and female, benefit from regular physical activity." Also, "significant health benefits can be obtained by including a moderate amount of physical activity on most, if not all, days of the week."

According to the Surgeon General's report, regular physical activity that is performed on most days of the week reduces the risk of developing or dying from some of the leading causes of illness and death in the United States. Regular physical activity improves health by

— reducing the risk of dying prematurely.
— reducing the risk of dying prematurely from heart disease.
— reducing the risk of developing diabetes.
— reducing the risk of developing high blood pressure.
— helping to reduce blood pressure in people who have high blood pressure already.
— reducing the risk of developing colon cancer.
— reducing feelings of depression and anxiety.
— helping to control weight.
— helping to build and maintain healthy bones, muscles, and joints.
— helping older adults become stronger and better able to move about without falling.
— promoting psychological well-being.

Regular physical activity should include cardiovascular exercise, resistance exercise (weight training), and flexibility exercise.

Total Personal Development

Total personal development includes physical, mental, social, emotional, and spiritual development.

Weight training can contribute to all of these areas of personal development in some way.

Physical

Weight training makes its most obvious contributions in the area of physical development. All of the following can be improved with a well planned weight training program:

- muscle strength
- tendon strength
- ligament strength
- bone strength
- muscle size
- muscle tone
- appearance
- posture
- flexibility
- metabolism
- joint stability
- muscle endurance
- power
- sports performance
- lean body mass
- physical fitness
- health

Weight training is a lifetime activity that can help you to maintain fitness, reduce body fat, and reduce the risk and rate of injury.

Mental

A successful weight training program requires: an understanding of how your body functions and responds to exercise, intelligent planning, consistent self-discipline, continual analysis, and insightful problem solving.

Social

Weight training is an activity that can be done alone, with one training partner, or with a group. Positive social qualities can be developed by doing weight training with others. Sharing, caring, encouraging, and helping are among the positive social behaviors that should occur during weight training workouts. These workouts provide a time to participate with others in an activity that produces positive results for all participants. In contrast to many recreational games, which must result in a winner and a loser, everyone is a winner in weight training.

Weight training provides a common activity in which to participate and a common topic to discuss, as well as a time to be together. It can be an excellent activity for family members or friends because everyone can be together, yet all can perform their own individual training program at their own level without interfering with anyone else's progress.

A good weight training program includes the achievement of goals. To share your goals with others, and to help others achieve their goals, is rewarding. A bond often develops among those who do difficult activities together.

Emotional

Weight training can help a person release emotional stress and tension. A measurable decrease in neuromuscular tension occurs following a weight training session. It also provides an opportunity to release anger and frustration in a socially acceptable and healthy manner — intense physical activity that is not directed at another person.

Because weight training involves overcoming physical challenges during each training session, some regular participants seem to adopt a more objective and positive approach to other challenges in their lives. This produces greater emotional stability.

Measurable and noticeable changes in physical appearance result from a well planned weight training program. Increased muscle size or muscle tone, or both, create a firm, shapely appearance for men and women alike. That firm, trim, athletic look never can be achieved by diet alone. Usually, posture also improves. These physical improvements tend to be accompanied by an enhanced self-image and greater self-esteem. Those who lift weights often look better and feel better about themselves.

Spiritual

The spirit refers to the soul or the life force within each living human. It is one of the intangible and invisible things in life that cannot be measured or adequately described. Yet, somehow you know it is there. It seems that those who increase the strength of their body and their mind also become stronger in spirit. They seem to have a greater resiliency, a greater life force, a stronger spirit.

It has been said that many can "talk the talk" but few can "walk the walk." Weight training can help you become a "can do" person instead of a "can't do" person.

PARTICIPATE IN YOUR OWN CREATION

You have an opportunity to participate in your own creation. The process of creation does not end with your birth, but continues throughout your life. All of the living cells in your body have a functional time limit. Millions of your cells are replaced every day. In terms of living cells you are not the same person you were last year, yesterday, or even an hour ago. You are in a continual process of changing, growing, becoming, and being created. What will you be like tomorrow, next week, or next year? Will you be better or worse than you are today?

Your attitude, behavior, and lifestyle choices have a significant impact on who you are and what you will become. Through weight training and healthy eating you begin by changing your body. However, you will find that as your body changes your life begins to change. I challenge you to follow a well-planned weight training program, and a healthy eating program, for one year and see for yourself. I believe after one year of disciplined weight training and eating you will see such a dramatic difference you will also believe in *weight training for life*.

Questions, Concerns, and Answers

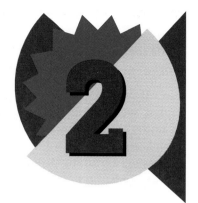

Can I just tone my muscles and not increase my muscle size?

Yes. By designing your training program so that you use moderate to light resistance (60% to 80% of your 1 repetition maximum) for relatively high repetitions (12 to 15 repetitions) and relatively few sets (1 or 2 sets) of relatively few exercises (1 exercise per muscle group) performed relatively few days per week (2 or 3 days per week), your strength and muscle tone will increase and you generally will experience little noticeable increase in muscle size. Actually, a lot of very hard work is necessary for most men and women to increase their muscle size.

If I build muscle, will it turn to fat when I stop weight training?

No. Muscle tissue and fat tissue are two distinctly different kinds of tissue in the human body, and muscle tissue cannot become fat tissue. If you stop training, however, you can accumulate more body fat.

Muscle tissue adapts to the demands placed upon it. When you stop training, your muscles will adapt to the new demand. If the new demand is much lower than it was before, the muscles will respond by getting smaller and weaker (*atrophy*). If you continue eating like you did when you were training hard every day, the extra calories now will be stored as body fat. Even if you manage to stay at the same body weight, you will have less muscle and more fat, leaving you with the outward appearance that your muscles have turned to fat.

Because fat tissue is not as dense as muscle tissue, you also can expect to gain inches in your body circumference measurements.

To make matters worse, as you lose metabolically active muscle tissue, your ability to use calories is reduced. Muscle cells are active calorie-burning cells. As these calorie-burning cells atrophy, your metabolic rate slows down and you need even fewer calories than before. To think you can maintain a trim, muscular, shapely appearance by diet alone is foolish. Are you beginning to realize the importance of *weight training for life*?

Are nutrition and rest important for weight training progress?

Yes. Weight training workouts provide a stimulus for positive changes to occur in your body, but without adequate nutrition and rest the changes may be very slow or may not occur at all. Your weight training workouts could be a waste of time if you do not eat and sleep properly. See Chapter 13 for more details on nutrition and rest.

Will weight training make a woman look masculine?

No. Hormones, not weight training, determine if a woman appears more masculine or more feminine. On the average, men have 6 to 10 times more testosterone than women. The higher levels of testosterone contribute to the secondary characteristics we generally consider as masculine. Women who train with weights generally develop healthy, shapely, trim female figures.

Will weight training make me muscle-bound?

No. If you follow correct weight training principles, weight training will not make you muscle-bound. "Muscle-bound" refers to a condition in which a person has a limited range of joint motion. One weight training principle is to train each muscle through a full range of motion. Each muscle should be exercised from full extension to full contraction. Also, the opposing muscles should receive an equal amount of exercise so the muscles on one side of a joint do not develop more than those on the other side. When these principles are followed, the weight trainer generally will experience an increase, rather than a decrease, in flexibility and joint mobility. The United States has many more "fat-bound" people than "muscle-bound" people.

Athletes may become muscle-bound as a result of the unbalanced muscular development induced by many sports. Also, when athletes train with weights to improve their sports performance, they typically train only those muscles that already are over-developed, and ignore balanced development. The result is that athletes sometimes see weight training as the reason for their muscle-bound condition when their condition actually is the result of a poorly planned weight training program.

The gymnast is probably one of the best examples of a high level of strength development accompanied by a high level of flexibility. Research also has shown that olympic weight lifters are among the most flexible athletes at the Olympic Games.

Will weight training shape up a specific part of my body?

Yes and no. Exercises for a specific body part will firm up weak, sagging muscles and may result in a trimmer appearance but will not effectively reduce excess body fat stored in that area.

The idea of losing body fat from a specific body part is known as *spot reduction*. Examples of spot reduction are sit-ups to lose fat from the abdomen and hip extensions to lose fat from the hips. Unfortunately, the research to date indicates that spot reduction does not work. To lose fat from a specific area requires a reduction in total body fat. This is best accomplished by reducing caloric intake and increasing caloric expenditure.

Is aerobic exercise the best way to lose excess body fat?

No. The best way to lose body fat is a combination of aerobic exercise, weight training, and healthy eating. Aerobic exercise is a good way to use calories and develop your cardiovascular system. Weight training is necessary to build muscle tissue, which increases your ability to use calories and reshape your body. Healthy eating is necessary to avoid excess calorie intake and ensure an adequate supply of the nutrients you need to rebuild your body. The combination of these three is the best way to lose body fat.

Weight training is an important component of the fat loss process. The increase in muscle tissue will help with fat loss by giving you more active muscle tissue that is capable of using calories and by increasing your resting metabolic rate so you will use more calories even when you are resting. If you want to improve the shape of your body you need to include *weight training for life*.

Will weight training make me slower?

No. Coaches used to tell their athletes not to lift weights because it would make them slower. The research in this area, however, indicates that the opposite is true: Weight training increases speed. Muscle contraction is responsible for human movement. With weight training, strength increases more than body weight, so the individual will have a greater strength-to-weight ratio. A stronger muscle can move a body part faster. Muscular weakness and excess body fat will make you slower.

Will weight training damage my joints?

No. Weight training exercises done correctly will increase joint strength. Exercises should be performed in a smooth, continuous manner.

Weight training exercises performed improperly could damage your joints. Jerking, throwing, and dropping weights should be avoided because these incorrect lifting techniques may result in injury.

What if I don't have time for weight training?

Everyone gets 168 hours a week, nobody gets more and nobody gets less. "Having time" is about prioritizing what is most important to you. If you don't have time for weight training you have either set your weight training goals too high (requiring too much time) or there are too many things in your life that you see as more important. Keep a time log for a week and see where you are spending time, investing time, and wasting time. According to a recent survey, the average American watches television 3 to 4 hours a day but doesn't have time to exercise.

Does weight training require hours of training each week?

No. Weight training is one of the most efficient forms of exercise. All of the major muscle groups in your body can be trained in 15 to 20 minutes two or three times each week. You will not find many effective exercise programs faster than that!

The amount of time you need to spend training with weights will be related to the goals you set for yourself. Body builders, olympic lifters, and power lifters do spend many hours each week training with weights; however, that is what they enjoy doing, and they have set some very high goals.

Will weight training ruin my coordination?

No. There is some neuromuscular adjustment to an increase in strength, but most people make this minor adjustment with no problem because strength gain is relatively slow. For the athlete in a sport in which "touch" or "timing" is critical, it is advisable to increase strength during the off-season and maintain that strength level through the competitive season. For the weak and untrained individual, weight training generally will improve coordination.

Can I gain as much strength from participating in sports as I can from weight training?

No. Most sports do not provide the right type, intensity, duration, or frequency of exercise to increase strength effectively. Weight training can produce a strength gain stimulus in one minute that is greater than a muscle would receive in hours of participation in most recreational activities.

Many recreational sports injuries are the result of placing an unfit body in a competitive situation. You should gain strength to participate in sports instead of participating in sports to gain strength.

Could heavy lifting cause a hernia?

Yes. A hernia, or a rupture in the abdominopelvic cavity, occurs when any of the internal organs is pushed through the wall that surrounds it. If you hold your breath and strain to lift an object that is too heavy, the pressure in the abdominal cavity increases to a high level and may result in a hernia. This often happens to individuals who do not train on a regular basis and do not know their own capability or correct lifting technique. The unfit person moving furniture is a classic example.

It is possible, but highly unlikely, that a hernia would occur during a well planned weight training program using correct lifting techniques. Correct weight training procedures require that you not hold your breath while lifting. Exhaling as you exert force is generally best. In weight training you should learn about, and practice, correct lifting mechanics and breathing techniques. These two factors, along with knowing how much weight you can lift safely, should reduce your risk of experiencing a hernia while weight training.

Hernias occur approximately 20 times less often among weight trainers than among non-weight trainers!

Can weight training develop total health-related physical fitness?

Yes. It is possible for a well planned circuit weight training program to develop all aspects of health-related physical fitness. Total health-related physical fitness involves the development of cardiovascular endurance, strength, muscular endurance, flexibility, and control of body fat. Most weight training programs, however, can best develop strength or muscular endurance. More effective ways are available to develop the other aspects of physical fitness.

Is weight training only for those who are young and athletic?

No. Weight training is a healthy lifetime fitness activity for males and females of all ages. Young athletes do use weight training to improve athletic performance, but that is certainly not the only use.

When is a person too old to start weight training?

Never. A person is never too old to start a sensible weight training program. Some people may be too unhealthy, but never too old. *Weight training for life* can be beneficial for anyone who has a muscular system to maintain. Each person should have an individualized training program. Your goals, training programs, and results will be different, but weight training can be beneficial at any age. Research has shown that individuals who are more than 90 years old gain strength and muscle mass when they begin lifting weights.

What if I miss a workout?

You will miss a workout sometime, everybody does. Just get back on your training schedule and keep going. Over a period of many years a few missed workouts will not make much difference. The worst thing you can do is quit. Quitting makes a big difference. Weight training is a lifetime fitness activity and the benefits come from years of regular training.

Why should I spend my time and energy lifting weights?

Most people lift weights to improve their appearance, health, and movement performance. *Weight training for life* can add more life to your years and maybe more years to your life.

Muscle Structure and Function

3

YOUR MUSCULAR SYSTEM

Your body has approximately 600 muscles, making up about 50% of your total body weight. Skeletal muscles account for about 40% of your total body weight, and the other 10% is primarily involuntary muscle of the circulatory and digestive system. Although muscles vary a great deal in size, shape, arrangement of fibers, and internal characteristics, they all perform the same general function — which is to provide movement. It is difficult to over-emphasize the importance of muscle tissue. All human movement is the result of muscle contraction.

CHARACTERISTICS OF MUSCLE TISSUE

Extensibility

Extensibility refers to the ability of muscle tissue to be stretched. If muscle tissue could not stretch, you would not have the mobility or range of motion that you now have.

Elasticity

Elasticity is the ability of muscle tissue to return to its normal resting length and shape after being stretched. If muscle tissue did not have elasticity, it would remain at whatever length you stretched it to.

Excitability

Excitability refers to the ability of muscle tissue to receive a stimulus from the nervous system.

Contractility

Contractility is the quality that really sets muscle tissue apart. When a stimulus is received, muscle tissue can contract, or shorten.

These four characteristics combine to make muscle tissue a very special kind of tissue. Muscle tissue is responsible for every movement your body makes.

TYPES OF MUSCLE TISSUE

Cardiac

Cardiac muscle is found only in the heart and is considered involuntary muscle because a person cannot consciously contract the heart muscle.

Smooth

Smooth muscle primarily lines hollow internal structures such as blood vessels and the digestive tract. Smooth muscle also is considered involuntary because its contraction and relaxation are automatic functions and not the result of conscious voluntary control.

Skeletal

The primary focus of this book is the development of skeletal muscle, which is attached to the bones or skeletal system. Skeletal muscle is voluntary muscle, and the contraction of skeletal muscle is a result of conscious voluntary control.

THE MUSCULOSKELETAL SYSTEM AS A LEVER SYSTEM

The three classifications of levers are: first class, second class, and third class. All three types of levers are found in the skeletal system of the human body. Not only are there three types of levers, but there are also six different kinds of joints that are considered freely movable. The result is a wide range of human movement possibilities. The movements that take place are the result of muscle tissue pulling on separate bones across a joint. Some joints, such as the ball-and-socket joint of the shoulder, have a wide range of movement possibilities that may be strengthened, whereas others, such as the hinge joint of the elbow, are limited to two movements, flexion and extension.

THE STRUCTURE OF SKELETAL MUSCLE

Each of your skeletal muscles has connective tissue through it and around it. Where this connective tissue attaches a muscle to a bone, it is called a *tendon*. The tendon is continuous with the connective tissue that encloses the muscle tissue.

The connective tissue that encloses skeletal muscle tissue is divided into three categories. *Epimysium* is connective tissue that surrounds the entire muscle. *Perimysium* is connective tissue that surrounds a fasciculus, or bundle of muscle fibers. *Endomysium* is connective tissue that surrounds a muscle fiber.

When you stretch a muscle, you are primarily stretching the connective tissue. It is important that the intensity of the stretch be sufficient to increase the length of the connective tissue without tearing it. Refer to Chapter 4 on stretching and flexibility for specific stretching guidelines.

Within the muscle are bundles of *muscle fibers* (muscle cells). Skeletal muscle fibers (cells) are generally long and relatively small in diameter. (See Figure 3.1.)

Within each muscle fiber are long thread-like structures called *myofibrils*. These myofibrils run lengthwise through the muscle fiber. Each myofibril consists of many *sarcomeres* attached end to end. See Figure 3.1. The sarcomere is the basic contractile unit of skeletal muscle tissue. (See Figures 3.1 and 3.2.) Within the sarcomere are *myofilaments*. The thinner myofilaments are called *actin*, and the thicker myofilaments are called *myosin*. According

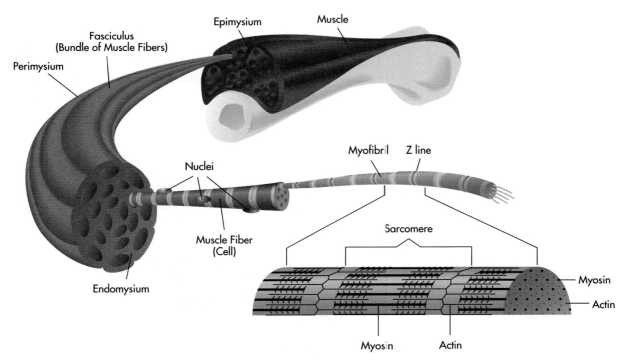

FIGURE 3.1   Components of skeletal muscle tissue.

to the sliding filament theory of muscle contraction, the myosin filaments have cross bridges that contact the actin filaments. The actin and myosin filaments do not change in length, but the myosin cross bridges pull the actin filaments toward the center of the sarcomere. Because the actin filaments are attached to the ends of the sarcomere, the sarcomere becomes shorter in length as the actin filaments are pulled toward the center. (See Figures 3.2 and 3.3.)

MUSCLE CONTRACTION AND EXERCISE MOVEMENTS

Muscle tissue can only contract or relax. Therefore, muscle can only pull on bones or stop pulling on bones. Muscle tissue cannot push. In some exercises an object, such as a barbell, is pushed away from the body. This is accomplished by muscles pulling on bones and causing the joints to extend. In other exercises muscles pull on bones to pull a weight toward the body. All exercises involve muscles pulling on bones across a joint. The movement that takes place depends upon the structure of the joint and the position of the muscle attachments involved. (See Figure 3.4.)

Isometric Contraction

Iso refers to equal, and *metric* refers to length or measure; therefore, an isometric contraction is one in which the muscle maintains an equal length. This occurs when contracting a muscle and creating a force against an immovable object. The muscle

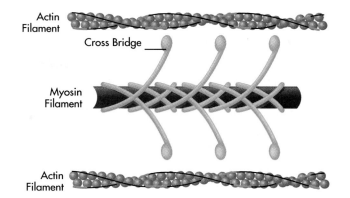

FIGURE 3.3 At higher magnification, during muscle contraction, cross bridges from the myosin attach to actin filaments and pull the actin filaments toward the center of the sarcomere.

contracts and tries to shorten but cannot overcome the resistance. An example of an isometric contraction is trying to lift a truck.

Isotonic Contraction

Tonic refers to tone or tension; therefore, an isotonic exercise is one in which movement occurs but muscle tension remains about the same. An example is a complete barbell curl.

Actually, during barbell and dumbbell exercises, while the external resistance remains constant, the muscle does not maintain constant tone throughout the exercise movement because of the continuous change in its angle of pull on the bone. Therefore, a new term is gaining some popularity in the research

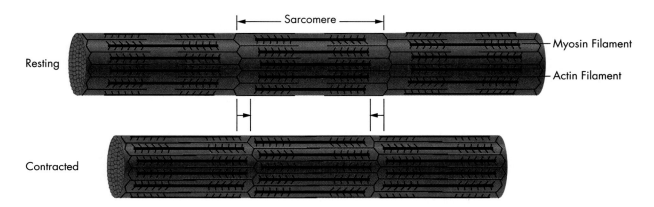

FIGURE 3.2 During muscle contraction, cross bridges from the myosin attach to actin filaments and pull the actin filaments toward the center of the sarcomere.

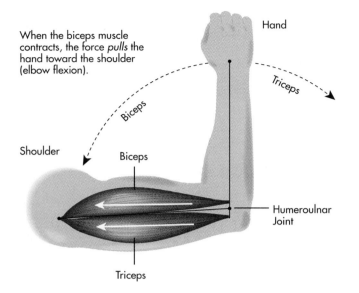

When the biceps muscle contracts, the force *pulls* the hand toward the shoulder (elbow flexion).

Hand

Triceps

Biceps

Shoulder

Biceps

Humeroulnar Joint

Triceps

When the triceps muscle contracts, the force *pulls* the hand away from the shoulder (elbow extension).

FIGURE 3.4 Two muscles showing pulling characteristics.

literature and may transfer to the popular literature. *DCER* stands for dynamic constant external resistance training. This is not a new type of training but, rather, an attempt to be more accurate in describing exercise movements against a constant external resistance, because the resistance, not the muscle tone, is what remains constant.

Concentric Contraction

A *concentric* contraction is a shortening contraction. The muscle becomes shorter and overcomes the resistance. An example is lifting the weight upward during the barbell curl.

Eccentric Contraction

An *eccentric* contraction is a lengthening contraction. The muscle contracts and tries to shorten but is overcome by the resistance. Eccentric contractions allow you to lower things smoothly and slowly. An example is lowering the weight in a smooth, controlled manner during the barbell curl.

Isokinetic Contraction

Kinetic refers to motion; therefore, a true isokinetic contraction is a constant speed contraction. The speed is set on the exercise device so the muscle can contract at 100% throughout the full range of motion without causing any acceleration. An example is the leg extension on a Cybex 350 Extremity Testing and Rehabilitation System.

MOTOR UNIT

A motor nerve is a nerve that comes from the brain or spinal cord and causes something to happen, contrasted with a sensory nerve, which takes information to the central nervous system. A motor unit consists of a single motor nerve and all the muscle fibers it sends impulses to. Although a motor nerve is connected to many muscle fibers, each muscle fiber is controlled by only one motor nerve. (See Figure 3.5.) A motor nerve that is responsible for very fine movement may be connected to very few muscle fibers, such as those responsible for eye movements. A motor nerve responsible for large or heavy human movements may be connected to many muscle fibers, such as those responsible for hip extension.

The All-or-None Principle

A muscle fiber contracts completely or not at all. If a stimulus for contraction is below the threshold value, no contraction occurs. If the stimulus is above the threshold value, complete contraction occurs. All of the muscle fibers in a motor unit contract completely or not at all. (See Figure 3.5.)

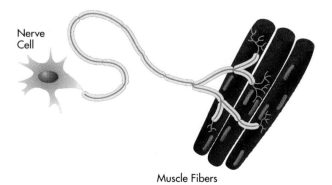

Nerve Cell

Muscle Fibers

FIGURE 3.5 Motor unit, composed of a motor nerve and muscle fibers.

Recruitment

Hundreds of motor units are contained in each muscle. The force a muscle exerts is determined primarily by the size and number of motor units recruited for a task.

As an example, refer to Figure 3.6. If a small amount of force is necessary, motor unit A may be used. In this case, three muscle fibers contract completely.

If a moderate amount of force is required, motor units A and B might both be used. In this case, seven muscle fibers contract completely.

Motor Nerves

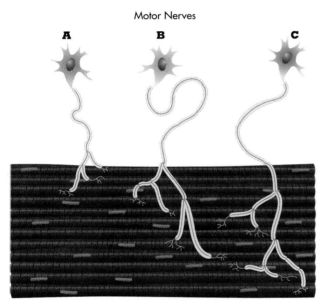

Muscle Fibers

FIGURE 3.6 Muscle fiber and motor unit recruitment.

If a maximum force is necessary, all three motor nerves may be activated, and they would stimulate 12 muscle fibers to contract completely, thus producing more force.

MUSCLE ATROPHY AND HYPERTROPHY

Muscles that are not used will shrink in size, or *atrophy* to a size that is adequate for the demands placed upon them. A good example of muscle atrophy occurs with a broken leg or arm that is immobilized in a cast during the bone healing process. When the cast is removed, that arm or leg is much smaller than the active arm or leg. The same thing happens to people who do not train their muscular system; however, the reduction in size occurs in both limbs and is so gradual that it often goes unnoticed.

The opposite is also generally true: Muscles that are forced to work harder than normal generally undergo *hypertrophy*, or an increase in size. This muscle growth is much more visible and more pronounced in men than it is in women. The reason for this greater increase in muscle size in men is thought to be related to the hormone testosterone, and to a larger number of muscle fibers in a muscle.

As your curiosity about muscle structure and function increases, you may want to refer to current human anatomy, human physiology, and exercise physiology textbooks for more detailed information.

Warm-Up, Flexibility, and Stretching

4

WARM-UP

Before participating in vigorous physical activity, most adults prefer to warm up. Warm-up activities usually consist of light muscular activity and some light stretching movements. A good warm-up will improve performance in weight training and should reduce the risk of injury.

One effective way to warm up for weight training is to perform light warm-up sets for each exercise before progressing to heavier sets for that same exercise. (See Figure 4.1.) For example, if your weight training program begins with bench press, you perform one or more sets of bench press slowly and smoothly to stretch and warm up the exact muscles and joints that will be used when you perform heavier sets of this same exercise. Almost all olympic lifters, power lifters, body builders, and athletes

warm up for heavy exercise in this manner. This method of warm-up seems to be beneficial for mental preparation as well as physical preparation to exert greater effort in later, heavier sets of an exercise.

Another effective way to warm up is to perform some type of cardiovascular activity before training with weights — activities such as walking, jogging, and bicycling.

FLEXIBILITY

Flexibility refers to the range of motion available in a joint. It is specific to each joint and each direction in which the joint allows movement. Therefore, a person might be flexible in shoulder joint movements and tight in hip joint movements. An individual also could be flexible in hip joint flexion but tight in hip joint extension or hyperextension.

Correct weight training should increase your flexibility. Correct weight training consists of (1) exercise through a full range of joint motion in a smooth and continuous manner, and (2) a balanced program of exercises for all opposing muscle groups that surround a joint.

Those who do not perform any exercise, those who participate in only one sport, and athletes who have trained with weights but have used partial movements or have neglected to develop opposing muscle groups are frequently less flexible than those who train correctly with weights.

How much flexibility is enough? No absolute measurable standard exists for how much flexibility you need to be healthy. In general, a joint should move freely in all of the directions appropriate for that joint.

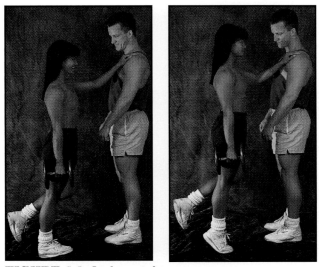

FIGURE 4.1 Light weight warm-up sets.

17

Is more flexibility better? Not always. There is a trade-off between flexibility and joint stability. If a joint has too much flexibility, it is less stable and the individual is more likely to experience dislocation-type injuries. On the other hand, if a joint has too little flexibility, it is very stable but the individual is more likely to experience soft tissue injuries to the muscles, tendons, and ligaments.

Weight training can be an ideal exercise to arrive at the optimal amount of flexibility because each joint should be moved through a full range of motion, which increases or maintains flexibility, and all of the muscles, tendons, and ligaments that surround and support a joint are strengthened by the progressive resistance. (See Figure 4.2.) One result of correct weight training should be strong, flexible joints.

Equipment can make a difference. Dumbbells generally allow the greatest range of motion and therefore may contribute more to flexibility. (See Figure 4.3.) The range of motion of some exercise machines is not as great as that of the individual using the machine. In this case, the individual will not increase flexibility when exercising on that particular machine.

STRETCHING

Stretching is a type of exercise used to increase flexibility. The range of motion of a joint is usually restricted by the soft tissue surrounding it — muscles, tendons, and ligaments. Therefore, stretching exercises should gently stretch these soft tissues without

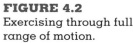

FIGURE 4.2
Exercising through full range of motion.

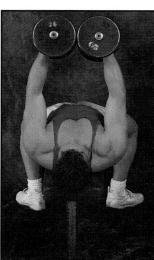

FIGURE 4.3
Using dumbbells to promote range of motion.

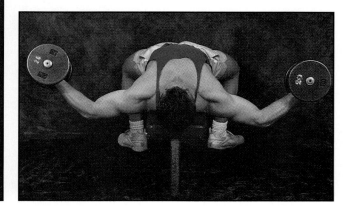

damaging them or the joint. The following guidelines have been proven to meet this criteria.

Type

Stretching exercises can be performed in different ways. *Static stretch* is a method of stretching in which the bones of a joint are moved to the point where the soft tissues surrounding the joint restrict further movement. These soft tissues (muscle, tendon, ligament, joint capsule) then are gently stretched and held in this stretched position for a period of time.

Six reasons for recommending static stretch are:

- It is an effective way to increase flexibility.
- The risk of injury is low.
- It is easy to learn.
- You can stretch alone.
- Static stretch relieves some types of muscle soreness.
- Performed correctly, static stretch does not cause muscle soreness (some other methods of stretching can cause muscle soreness).

Intensity

To be effective in increasing flexibility, the soft connective tissue surrounding a joint has to be stretched to a position about 10% beyond its normal length. This is difficult to measure. However, we have a built-in mechanism for judging the intensity of a static stretching exercise: pain receptors.

When you are stretching at the correct intensity, you will experience moderate discomfort in the muscles being stretched. If the muscles do not have enough tension for you to tell which muscles are being stretched, you have not stretched far enough. On the other hand, if you experience pain while stretching, you are going too far and could injure yourself.

Duration

When you are performing static stretching exercises, you should hold a static position at an intensity of moderate discomfort for at least 10 seconds but not more than 30 seconds. You should perform each stretching exercise at least once. For the average person who is stretching for physical fitness, performing each stretching exercise more than three times is not necessary.

Frequency

To be most effective in increasing flexibility, static stretching exercises should be repeated at least 3 days per week. Static stretching exercises can be performed up to 7 days per week.

JOINTS TO STRETCH

A stretching exercise can be designed for every muscle and every joint in your body; however, stretching the following major areas is more practical: shoulders, wrists, hips, knees, and ankles. Each of these joints is stretched in each major direction that it can move, and held in that position for 10 to 30 seconds. Your weight training instructor can give you advice on safe stretching exercises.

Recently, many good stretching exercises have been labeled as potentially harmful. Generally, it is not the exercise itself but, instead, the way the exercise is performed that makes it harmful. You always should be careful when stretching so the exercises produce flexibility and not injury.

WHEN TO STRETCH

Many individuals feel better if they stretch their muscles and joints prior to more vigorous exercise such as weight training. This stretching may help prevent exercise injuries and may improve performance, though little conclusive research evidence is available to support either of these common beliefs.

Some research has indicated that vigorous stretching of cold muscles may be harmful. Therefore, any stretching before warming the muscles should be done carefully. Stretching cold muscles should be done through light, gentle stretching exercises designed to loosen up the movements of those joints.

Vigorous stretching to increase flexibility should be done only after the muscles and joints are thoroughly warmed up. One good time to do this type of stretching is immediately after your weight training workout. Another good time to stretch is during the rest between sets.

STRETCHING GUIDELINES

Type:	Static stretch
Intensity:	Moderate discomfort
Duration:	10- to 30-second hold 1 to 3 repetitions
Frequency:	3 to 7 days per week

Safe and Effective Weight Training

MEDICAL CLEARANCE

It is a good idea to have a complete physical examination before starting any new exercise program. Tell your physician you want to start a weight training program and ask if there is any reason you should not. Medical clearance becomes more important as you get older, if you are overweight, or if you have not participated in a physical training program for a long time.

CLOTHING

Clothing for weight training should allow freedom of movement during all exercises through a complete range of motion. See Figure 5.1 for examples of appropriate clothing for weight training. When the weather or the gym is warm, most weight trainers wear gym shorts, a t-shirt or tank-top, socks and shoes. When the training environment is cold, a cotton sweatsuit is usually worn over the shorts

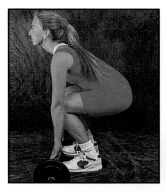

FIGURE 5.1
Appropriate clothing to wear while weight training.

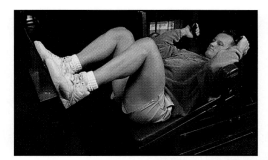

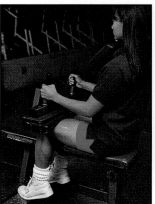

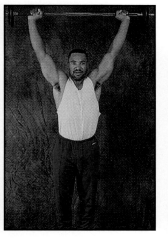

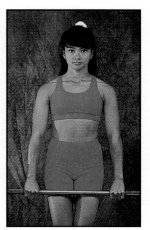

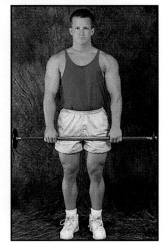

and shirt. Cotton material absorbs perspiration better than most synthetic materials and tends to be more comfortable during exercise. However, many new exercise clothing materials and styles work just as well.

The clothing you select for weight training should be comfortable, durable, and it should help keep your muscles warm while training. In addition, you should look good and feel good about your appearance when you are weight training. If you don't feel good about yourself during an activity, the human tendency is to quit participating in the activity.

Wear shoes when training with weights. The weight room has many hard objects you might kick, drop, or step on.

PERFORMING A WEIGHT TRAINING EXERCISE

The following are guidelines for performing a weight training exercise to maximize your weight training progress and your safety.

Strict Exercise Form

By maintaining strict exercise form (see Figure 5.2), you will keep the load on the muscles that the exercise was designed to develop. When you do not maintain strict exercise form, you will reduce the load on the muscles you are trying to develop and will increase your risk of injury.

Smooth Movement

Don't exercise with a jerk. Weight training exercises should be performed in a smooth, continuous movement. Some exercises are done faster than others, and some involve acceleration, but they should all be smooth. This allows the muscle to apply force to the resistance throughout the full range of motion. The purpose of weight training is to build healthy muscle tissue, not to tear it apart.

Full Range of Motion

Whenever possible, a muscle should be exercised from full extension to full contraction and back to

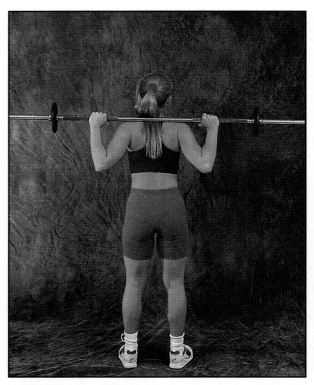
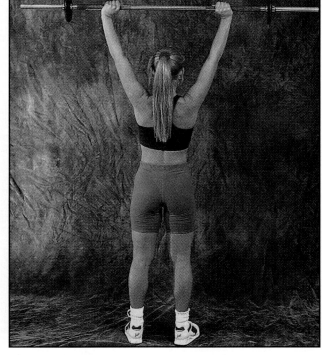

FIGURE 5.2 Maintain strict exercise form when lifting weights.

full extension (see Figure 5.3). This results in strength gains throughout the complete range of motion of the muscle in the concentric phase (shortening) and the eccentric phase (lengthening). It also helps improve flexibility.

Concentric Phase

In the concentric phase of an exercise, the muscle contraction overcomes the resistance. This causes the muscle to get shorter as the weight is raised. For most exercises this concentric phase should take 1 to 2 seconds.

Eccentric Phase

During the eccentric phase of an exercise, the same muscles that raised the weight now lower the weight. In this phase the weight is allowed to overcome the force of muscle contraction. Therefore, even though the muscle is contracting and trying to shorten, it is being lengthened by the pull of the resistance. Eccentric contractions allow us to lower objects in a smooth, controlled manner. Weights should be lowered smoothly and continuously.

The eccentric phase of an exercise should take at least as long as the concentric phase (1 to 2 seconds), and sometimes up to twice as long (2 to 4 seconds). Because the same muscles are working to raise and lower the weight, only half an exercise would be completed by allowing the weight to drop after it has been lifted.

Among those who gain the least from a weight training exercise are those who throw the weight upward using poor exercise form, incorrect muscle groups, and momentum. Then, once the weight has been raised, they allow it to drop back to the starting position. Those individuals may move more weight, but their muscles receive less benefit from the exercise and they have a much greater risk of injury.

Breathing

A good general rule for breathing during weight training exercises is to exhale during the greatest exertion — usually the concentric phase of the exercise (lifting) — and inhale when lowering (the eccentric phase). One exception to this rule occurs when performing overhead pressing movements. Some weight trainers are more comfortable inhaling as they press the weight overhead and exhaling as they lower it.

Proper breathing is an important part of correct exercise technique. It should be practiced with lighter weights while new exercises are being learned. A

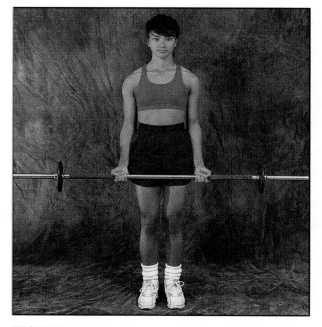
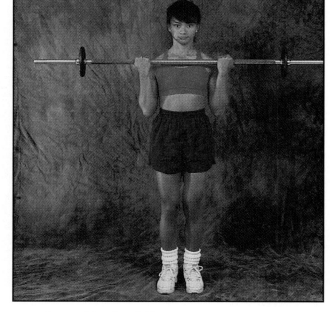

FIGURE 5.3 Exercise muscles from full extension to full contraction and back to full extension.

breathing pattern should be learned with each exercise. There is some room for individual differences and preferences.

The one thing that should be avoided is holding your breath while straining to lift a heavy weight. This produces a great deal of pressure inside the chest cavity and the abdominal cavity, making it difficult, or even impossible, for the blood in the veins to return to the heart. The sudden high pressure caused by straining to lift a heavy weight while holding your breath could cause dizziness, a blackout, a stroke, a heart attack, or a hernia. Although events such as these are extremely rare in weight trainers, the possibility of their occurrence should emphasize the importance of learning to breathe properly during the exercises.

Concentration

Full attention should be focused on the muscles that are moving the weight (Figure 5.4). This concentration should be maintained on every repetition, and throughout every set, to gain the maximum benefit from the exercise. Weight trainers should not let their mind wander while performing a weight training exercise.

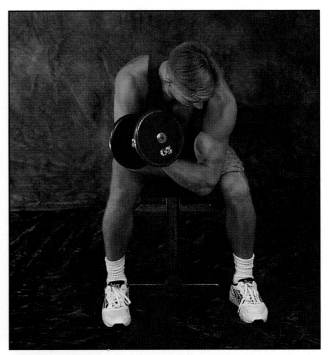

FIGURE 5.4 Focusing full attention on muscles moving the weight.

Isolated Intensity

Isolated intensity is closely related to concentration and getting the greatest benefit from weight training in the least amount of exercise time. Isolated intensity means focusing on a muscle, or group of muscles, that you wish to develop and forcing the muscle to work very hard. As you advance in your muscle training, you will learn how to force a muscle to work to temporary failure. This is beyond the point where you would like to quit and to the point where the muscle cannot perform the task. It is very intense exercise for an isolated group of muscles and is much more effective in producing gains than easier sets that are stopped when they begin to get difficult.

Working muscles to the point of temporary muscular failure is not recommended for beginning weight trainers. It can result in extreme muscle soreness and serious injury.

ADDITIONAL CONSIDERATIONS FOR MACHINE EXERCISES

All of the guidelines for performing a weight training exercise apply to the use of weight training machines as well; however, a few additional considerations will make the use of weight machines safe and effective.

Correct Body Position

Position yourself on the machine so the pivot point of your body, the correct joint for the exercise movement, is lined up with the pivot point of the machine (see Figure 5.5 and Figure 5.6). For example, if you are on an arm curl machine, your elbow joint should be lined up with the pivot point of the arm curl machine. Most machines are designed to fit a wide range of body sizes. The adjustments are usually for height. Make sure you have adjusted the machine for correct body position and all adjustments are locked in place before you attempt to lift.

Seat Belts

Several weight training machines have a seat belt to hold you on the machine and in the correct body position (Figure 5.6). Be sure to use the seat belt. It will make the exercise more effective and safer.

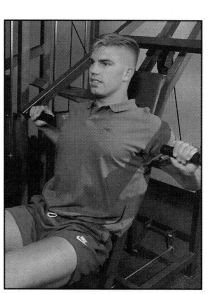

FIGURE 5.5
Maintain correct body position on machines.

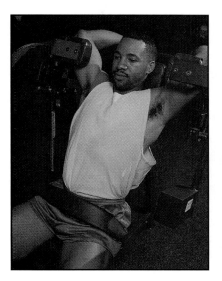

FIGURE 5.6
Seat belts on training machine.

may also cause the cable or chain to jump off the pulley. At the very least it will drop with a jerk, dramatically increasing the load on your muscles, tendons, ligaments, and joints.

Raise and lower the weight in a smooth controlled manner. If you allow the weight to drop after lifting it you may break a plate in the weight stack, the cable, the chain, or one of the pulleys.

Control the speed of movement on weight machines. Lifting the weight usually should take about 2 seconds, and lowering the weight should take 2 to 4 seconds. The weights should return gently and quietly to the weight stack. If you cannot control the speed of the weight, it is too heavy for you at this time. If you decrease the weight and perform the exercise correctly, you will get more benefit and faster gains. Also, your machine will last much longer.

Full Range of Motion

Most weight machines are designed to allow you to lift through the full range of joint motion. You would be wise to do it. You will develop strength through the full range of motion, get better muscle development, and maintain a reasonable amount of flexibility. See Figure 5.7.

Immediate Repairs

Like all machines, exercise machines have to be properly maintained. If you start to use a machine and find something that needs to be tightened or

Speed of Movement

Most machines are not designed for speed and power training. Speed and momentum can cause problems. First, you are more likely to injure yourself by lifting in a fast, jerky motion. Second, you are more likely to damage the machine by lifting too fast.

Many machines have weight stacks, pulleys, cables, and chains. If you lift the weight stack too quickly, it will gain momentum and may continue upward at the end of the lift, causing the weight stack to bang against the top of the machine. This

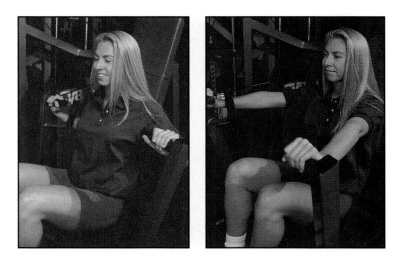

FIGURE 5.7 Using full range of motion.

adjusted, do it, or report it immediately. It generally takes only a few turns of a screwdriver or wrench and a few seconds to make it right. However, if you let it go and something breaks, it generally will be much more costly in time and money to get it repaired. Don't misuse weight machines, and do your part to keep them working properly. They will give you years of good lifting.

Keep Machines Clean

If many people use the same machines, it is courteous and thoughtful to carry a towel with you during your workout and wipe your perspiration off of the machine when you are finished with the exercise. It takes only a second or two and makes it much nicer for the next lifter.

Moving Parts

Maintain a safe distance from an exercise machine that is being used. Keep your hands and fingers away from moving weight stacks, cables, chains, levers, and pulleys.

TRAINING PARTNER

A good training partner can be your greatest asset. (See Figure 5.8.) A bad training partner can be your greatest liability. A good training partner makes training safer by being ready to spot on hazardous exercises so you can train to the limit of your capacity without fear of injury. A bad training partner is never ready when you need a spotter or is not paying attention during your exercises. A good training partner is always ready to help you load weights, change weights, and move equipment. A bad training partner lets you do all the work of setting up for exercises. A good training partner offers positive motivation and encouragement. A bad training partner maintains a negative attitude that dampens your enthusiasm. A good training partner is on time for every training session. A bad training partner frequently skips workouts or arrives late.

Even though you can make your best weight training progress with a good training partner, you still can make excellent progress training alone. A bad training partner can hinder your weight training progress. If your partner is unwilling or unable

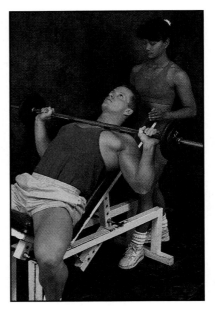

FIGURE 5.8
Training partner.

to change, you should train alone or find a new training partner. You also should be prepared to listen, as you may hear about some of your own faults as a training partner.

SPOTTING

When lifting weights, especially free weights, there are some exercises in which you could get pinned under a weight if you could not complete the exercise movement. For safety, and to get the maximum benefit from the exercise, you should always be spotted on these lifts. A spotter is a person who is in a position to help you complete the lift if it becomes necessary (See Figures 5.9 and 5.10).

Communication

Effective communication is the key to effective spotting. Before the lift, the lifter and spotter should talk briefly. Both the lifter and the spotter should know what exercise will be performed, how many repetitions will be attempted, how much help the lifter expects, if there will be any forced reps or negative reps at the end of the set, if the lifter expects help getting the weight into position (lift off), and if the lifter expects help guiding the weight back onto a rack at the end of the set. This communication before the lift takes only a few seconds and is time well spent. It significantly increases safety and reduces misunderstandings.

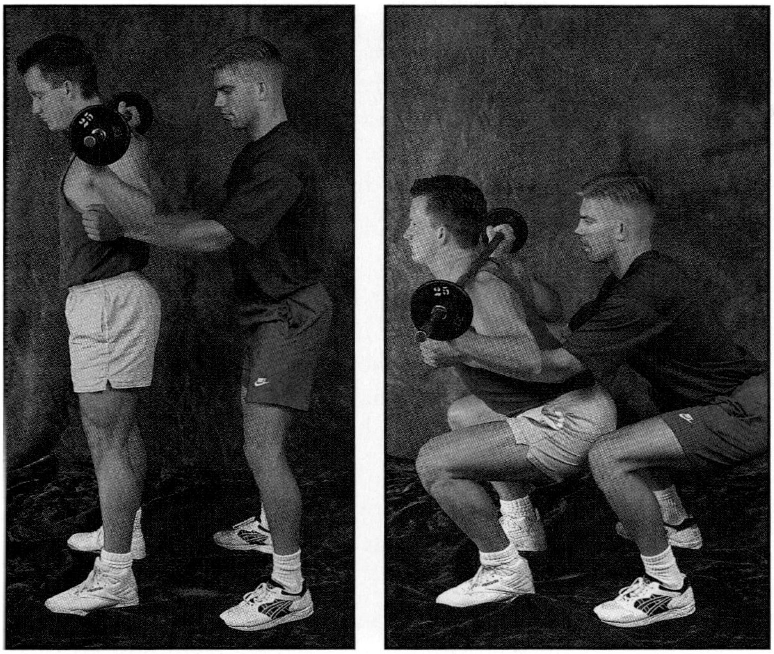

FIGURE 5.9 Spotting.

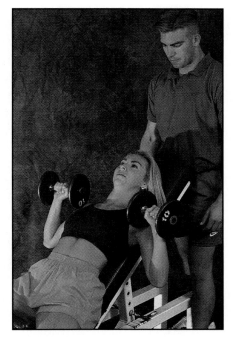

FIGURE 5.10 Stay alert! Give your full attention to spotting.

General Guidelines for Spotters

1. Be sure you are strong enough to help with the weight being attempted. If not, tell the lifter and try to find more help.

2. Be sure you know how the lifter expects to be spotted. If you are not sure, ask the lifter before the lift is attempted.

3. Be sure you know what signs or signals the lifter will use to communicate during the lift. Know what words and gestures the lifter will use to let you know what to do.

4. Stay alert! Give your full attention to spotting the lift. Do not look away from the lifter. Do not be distracted. Do not carry on a conversation with someone else during the lift.

5. Do not touch the bar during the exercise if the lifter can complete the lift without your help. By doing so, you may decrease the overload stimulus the lifter needs to make the desired gains.

6. Check the bar before the lift for balanced loading and secure collars.

7. Move weight plates or anything else near your feet that might cause you to trip or lose your balance.

8. Stay in a proper spotting and lifting position throughout the attempt so you are ready immediately if help is needed.

9. Do not jerk the bar away from the lifter or throw it off balance. Gently provide the amount of help needed to complete the lift.

10. Be a responsible spotter. The lifter is depending on you to do the job right.

General Guidelines for Lifters Being Spotted

1. It is your responsibility to make sure the spotter knows what you expect. Don't assume the spotter can read your mind. If the spotter did not do what you were expecting, it was your fault for getting under the bar without communicating clearly before the lift.

2. Don't quit on a repetition. Even if you cannot complete a repetition by yourself, keep trying and it should take very little lifting by the spotter to help you complete the lift. *Never* let go of the bar or quit on a lift when the spotter touches the bar.

3. Thank your spotter after each set.

SAFETY

The following are guidelines for safe weight training.

1. Move carefully and slowly in the weight room. The weight lifting area is not a good place for sudden, unexpected movements. Always be alert for movement around you. Do not back up without looking first. Watch where you are going.

2. Stay clear of other lifters and spotters. Avoid collisions with people and equipment.

3. Stay clear of weight machines when someone is lifting or in position to lift.

4. Fix broken equipment immediately, or set it aside, or put a sign on it. Do not attempt to use broken equipment.

5. Make sure you are in a stable position before you attempt a lift.

6. Use collars on all plate loading equipment such as barbells and dumbbells.

7. Perform all lifts using strict exercise form.

8. Do not hold your breath and strain to lift a weight.

9. Warm up and stretch before lifting.

10. Don't lift when you are sick. You are not likely to make much progress, and you expose everyone in the weight room to the same illness.

11. Don't fool around in the weight room. The weight lifting area is no place for practical jokes or wild behavior. Serious injuries can result from thoughtless and foolish behavior during weight training.

12. Do not twist your body, arch your back, or arch your neck while attempting to complete a lift.

13. Lift within your ability. Do not try to lift more weight than you can handle safely.

14. Adjust each machine to put you in the correct lifting position before starting a set.

15. Do not bounce weights off your body or off a weight stack. If you must bounce a weight to lift it, the weight is too heavy.

16. Be very careful when loading and unloading barbells that are resting on a rack. If you get too much weight on one end of a barbell, it will flip off the rack. This is a dangerous but common mistake by beginning lifters. Add and remove weight from each end of the bar as evenly as possible, keeping the bar balanced on the rack.

17. Store all weight training equipment properly. Do not leave it lying around on the floor. All dumbbells, barbells, and weight plates should have storage racks where the lifter will put them after completing the exercise.

18. Always control the speed and direction of the lift. If you cannot control the lift, the weight is too heavy. Reduce the weight and perform the lift correctly.

19. Do not perform lifts where you could be trapped under the weight without spotters who know what to do. (See Figure 5.11.)

20. Always be polite, courteous, and helpful in the weight room. This will create a safer and more pleasant training environment for everyone.

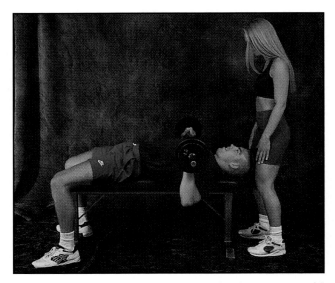

FIGURE 5.11 Do not perform a lift where you could be trapped under the weight unless you have a spotter.

A Beginning Weight Training Program

FREE WEIGHTS AND MACHINES

One beginning weight training program is presented in this chapter. Basic exercises are listed for free weights and machines. You will need to choose which you will use based on your preference and what is available to you.

Beginners often ask which is "better" — free weights or machines. The answer depends on several factors. The following are some of the factors to consider as you decide what is best for you.

Advantages of Machines

1. Machines are generally safer because you cannot get trapped under the weight. This is a real advantage if you will be training without a spotter.
2. Changing from one weight to another is faster because you only need to move a selector pin to the new weight. This is a great advantage if you choose to spend less time exercising.
3. Learning the exercise movement is easier and faster because the direction of the movement is controlled by the machine.

Advantages of Free Weights (Barbells and Dumbbells)

1. Free weights offer a greater variety of exercise movements than machines because they are free to move in any direction.
2. Free weights are available at a much lower cost than most exercise machines.

3. Free weights are easier to move from one location to another.
4. One size fits all. Adjustable barbells and dumbbells are the right size for almost everyone.
5. Additional stabilizing and assisting muscles are used to hold your body in the correct exercise position, keep the weight moving along the correct path, and balance the weight.

GRIPS

The grip on the barbell or exercise machine involves the position of the hands on the bar and the spacing of the hands.

Hand Position

There are three basic hand positions; pronated, supinated, and mixed. The *pronated grip* (thumbs toward each other) is also referred to as the overhand grip, overgrip, overgrasp, and regular grip. (See Figure 6.1.) The *supinated grip* (thumbs away from each other) is also referred to as the

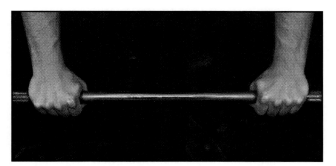

FIGURE 6.1 Pronated grip (overgrip).

underhand grip, undergrip, undergrasp, and reverse grip. (See Figure 6.2.) The *mixed grip* (one thumb toward the other hand and one thumb away from the other hand) is also referred to as the combined grip, alternate grip, and dead lift grip. (See Figure 6.3.)

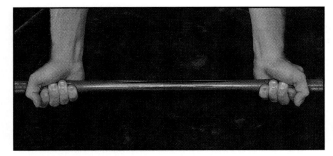

FIGURE 6.2 Supinated grip (undergrip).

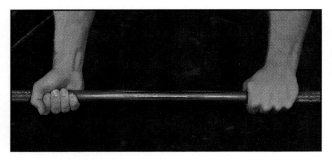

FIGURE 6.3 Mixed grip.

Always wrap your thumb around the bar for safety. Performing lifts where the bar is over your body and your thumbs are not around the bar is very risky and is not recommended. Also, do not lock your thumb around the bar and under your fingers. This hand position places your thumb in a position where injury is very likely.

Hand Spacing

There are three basic choices for hand spacing on the bar. The first is the regular or normal hand spacing in which your hands are placed on the bar approximately shoulder width apart. (See Figure 6.4.)

Some exercises are more effective with a narrow grip. The hands are closer together than shoulder width, normally 4 to 8 inches apart. (See Figure 6.5.)

Some exercises are more effective with a wide grip. The hands are placed on the bar at a distance that is wider than shoulder width. (See Figure 6.6.)

When you are learning a new exercise, first try the hand spacing that is recommended or illustrated in the exercise section of this book. Later, when you are more comfortable with the exercise movement, use a lighter weight and experiment with different hand spacings to find the ones that are most comfortable for you and the ones where you feel you get the greatest development for the muscles.

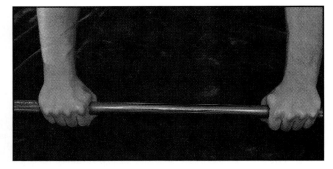

FIGURE 6.4 Shoulder-width grip.

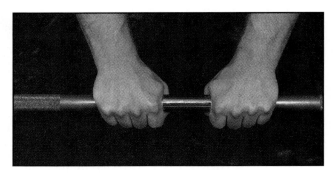

FIGURE 6.5 Narrow grip.

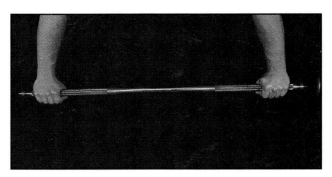

FIGURE 6.6 Wide grip.

BASIC LIFTS

Dead Lift

If you choose to lift with barbells and dumbbells, you frequently will need to lift the bar from the floor to assume the exercise position. There is a correct and an incorrect way to lift. Every time you lift a weight from the floor, use correct dead lift form, no matter how light the weight. You can injure your lower back by lifting improperly, and once injured, the low back does not tend to recover quickly or completely. Therefore, it is important to avoid injury to your back in the first place.

If you are lifting the weight from the floor into the starting exercise position, you will need to use the proper grip for the exercise to be performed instead of the mixed grip that is used most commonly when performing the dead lift as an exercise. For example, if you are picking up the bar to perform barbell arm curls, grasp the bar with an undergrip, then perform the dead lift as described to get into the starting position for the exercise.

DEAD LIFT

Muscles developed: Erector spinae, gluteus maximus, quadriceps, trapezius, rhomboids.

Starting position: Bend over and assume a mixed grip on a barbell that is lying on the floor; bend your knees and hips so that the hips are approximately knee level; keep your back flat.

Concentric phase: Keep your neck and back flat while straightening the hips and knees to arrive at a standing position.

Eccentric phase: Keep your neck and back flat as you slowly lower the weight back to the floor by bending your knees and hips.

Additional information: Extremely heavy weight can be handled in this exercise. Progress slowly, and maintain correct lifting position. Progressing too quickly or using improper lifting technique may result in injury.

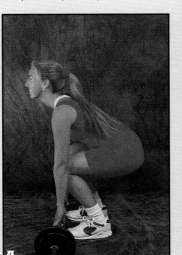
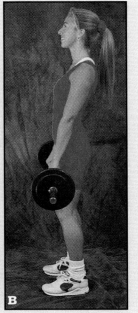

Clean

For some free weight exercises, such as the overhead press, you will need to get the weight to shoulder level to start the exercise. If a shoulder-height rack is available, you can lift the weight from the rack. If a rack is not available, you will need to lift the weight from the floor to your shoulders. This lift is called a clean. When you clean a weight, keep your back flat and lift with your legs. The proper body position for the pull on the clean is the same as the pull on the dead lift. Keep your back flat and lift with your legs.

The clean is used by more advanced lifters as an exercise. It is not generally recommended for beginners as an exercise unless they have excellent instruction and supervision.

BEGINNING EXERCISES

All of the exercises suggested for the beginning program are described in the exercise portion of this book. One exercise for each major muscle group or joint action is recommended for beginning weight trainers. During the first year or two of training, one exercise per body part will produce good results. Those who are weight training to develop physical fitness usually do not need more than one exercise per body part; however, it is a good idea to occasionally change the exercise you are performing to develop that body part.

More people have gained more muscle on simple weight training programs consisting of basic exercises than all of the complex and complicated programs combined.

CLEANS

Muscles developed: Trapezius, erector spinae, gluteus maximus, quadriceps.

Starting position: Bend over and grasp a barbell that is on the floor, with your hands approximately shoulder-width apart and in a pronated (thumbs in) grip; bend your knees and hips, keeping your head in line with your body, with your neck and back flat.

Concentric phase: Inhale as you lift the bar from the floor and accelerate the bar upward, gaining speed as it rises to the highest position to which you can pull it. The pull should continue upward to the level of your chest or shoulders. As the bar nears its highest point, quickly rotate your arms under the bar and bend your knees, catching the bar on your shoulders. Straighten your legs to a standing position and exhale.

Eccentric phase: Inhale and quickly rotate the arms from under the bar. Bend your arms, legs, and hips to decelerate the bar to a hang position with the bar resting against the upper thighs. Then slowly bend the knees and hips to lower the bar back to the floor. Exhale.

Variations:

1. Start with the weight up on blocks.
2. Start with the weight in a hang position (hang cleans).

Additional information: Keep your back straight. Do not jerk the weight from the floor, but lift and accelerate the weight.

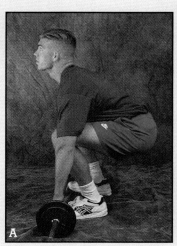

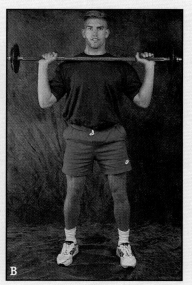

RECOMMENDED EXERCISES FOR BEGINNERS

Exercise Description	Free Weights	Machines
Chest (Chapter 7)	Barbell Bench Press	Prone or Seated Chest Press
Back (Chapter 8)	One Dumbbell Rowing	Seated or Low Pulley Rowing
Shoulders (Chapter 9)	Military Press	Seated Shoulder Press
Arms (Chapter 10)	Barbell Curl	Arm Curl
Legs (Chapter 11)	Squat One Dumbbell Calf Raise	Leg Press Calf Raise or Calf Press
Abdominals (Chapter 12)	Abdominal Crunches	Ab Machine Crunches
Back Extension (Chapter 12)	Back Extension	Back Extension

Above are basic exercises recommended for beginners.

FREQUENCY AND RESISTANCE

The exercises above should be performed three times each week with at least 48 hours of rest between training sessions. Start light, and progress slowly. If you are just starting a weight training program, you should begin with very light weight and learn to do each exercise with correct technique before you add resistance. Then, gradually add weight, but never at the cost of losing correct lifting technique. Ask your training partner or instructor to watch you perform each lift, and compare your technique with the photographs and descriptions in the exercise sections of this book. If you want to see yourself, have someone videotape your lifts so you can critique them yourself. Some weight training instructors like to grade students on correct lifting technique.

Weight training can be one of the most intense forms of exercise you will ever perform. Muscles can be isolated and worked extremely hard within a minute or two without experiencing total body fatigue. Therefore, beginners tend to overtrain and experience extreme delayed-onset muscle soreness during the next 2 or 3 days. This tendency to overtrain is also a product of the false belief, "If a little is good, more must be better." This is not always the case with weight training.

Beginners can easily overtrain the muscles to the point that they cannot recover before the next training session. The result is a decrease in performance and no gain.

The program suggested in this chapter is recommended for healthy young people of high school and college age (approximately 15 to 22 years old) who are near their peak of physical growth and who have been physically active. If you are older, or if you have been inactive for a long time, progress more slowly. Weight training is a lifetime activity. Progress slowly and safely. Avoid the injuries and extreme soreness that result from trying to add resistance too quickly.

THE FIRST SIX WEEKS

What is most important during the first few weeks of a weight training program? Safety and correct exercise technique. Use light weights and learn to perform each exercise in your program correctly. Learn the breathing pattern that works best and develop a habit of breathing correctly during your exercises.

Allow your body to gradually adapt to this new demand. Progress slowly to keep muscle soreness to a minimum. Learn to focus your concentration on the muscles being developed during each repetition of each exercise.

Weeks 1 and 2 (1 × 20)

For the first 2 weeks (6 exercise sessions), perform each exercise once (one set), completing 20 exercise movements (20 repetitions) in that set. Example: Bench Press: 1 set of 20 repetitions (1 × 20).

If you complete all 20 repetitions while maintaining correct exercise technique, you may increase the resistance for the next training session. If a weight feels very light and the repetitions are extremely easy, a large increase in the weight could be made for the next training session. If a weight feels moderately difficult, a small increase should be made for the next training session. By the end of 2 weeks (6 training sessions), you should be training with a weight that makes it difficult for you to complete 20 repetitions while maintaining correct lifting technique.

If you complete at least 15 repetitions, but fewer than 20, use the same resistance for your next training session and try to increase the number of repetitions completed.

If you complete fewer than 15 repetitions, reduce the resistance for your next training session.

Any time you begin to use incorrect lifting technique to move the weight, stop after that repetition and either use a lighter weight and repeat the set or schedule a lighter weight for the next training session. Proper exercise form should not be sacrificed to complete repetitions. When you can no longer perform repetitions correctly, stop the set and record the number of repetitions you performed correctly.

Weeks 3 and 4 (1 × 20) (1 × 10)

During the next 2 weeks (6 training sessions) perform 1 set of 20 repetitions (1 × 20), followed by 1 set of 10 repetitions (1 × 10). Keep trying to find the heaviest weight you can lift 20 times on the first set.

After resting 1 or 2 minutes, perform 1 set of 10 repetitions. Each time you complete 10 repetitions in the second set, schedule a heavier weight for the next exercise session. Following this procedure, gradually work toward the heaviest weight you can lift 20 times in the first set and the heaviest weight you can lift 10 times in the second set while maintaining strict exercise form. If you cannot complete at least 8 repetitions in the second set, reduce the resistance for the next training session.

Weeks 5 and 6 (1 × 20) (1 × 10) (1 × 5)

During weeks 5 and 6 (the next 6 workouts), perform 1 set of 20 repetitions (1 × 20) first, 1 set of 10 repetitions (1 × 10) second, and 1 set of 5 (1 × 5) third. Continue to search *safely* for the heaviest weight you can handle in each set.

If you complete 5 good repetitions in the third set, schedule a heavier weight for the next training session. If you complete at least 3 repetitions in the third set, keep the weight and try to increase your reps. If you can not complete at least 3 good repetitions, reduce the weight for the next training session.

GUIDELINES FOR PRODUCTIVE TRAINING

After this first 6 weeks of training, you should have had time to develop a good foundation of total body strength and time to finish reading this book so that you are able to plan your own weight training programs based on goals you have set for yourself. You should also be able to plan a method of record keeping and measuring your progress toward your goals. Some overall guidelines are:

1. Perform each repetition with correct technique and complete concentration.
2. Make gradual, but consistent, increases in exercise intensity.
3. Complete each scheduled training session. Form the habit of never missing a scheduled training session.
4. Maintain a positive attitude. Enjoy each training session.
5. Eat right. Healthy eating is critical to optimal weight training progress.
6. Get enough rest. Weight training serves only as a stimulus for positive changes to take place in your body. The changes are biological adaptations that actually occur between exercise sessions. Without adequate nutrition and rest, it is difficult for these positive changes to take place.
7. Stay healthy. You may not normally think of this as a choice, but your health is closely related to your lifestyle. Make healthy choices.

Name_____ Section_____

Date												
Exercise	Wt	Rep	Wt	Rep	Wt	Rep	Wt	Rep	Wt	Rep	Wt	Rep

Name_____ Section_____

Date												
Exercise	Wt	Rep	Wt	Rep	Wt	Rep	Wt	Rep	Wt	Rep	Wt	Rep

Name_____ Section_____

Date												
Exercise	Wt	Rep	Wt	Rep	Wt	Rep	Wt	Rep	Wt	Rep	Wt	Rep

Name_____ Section_____

Date												
Exercise	Wt	Rep	Wt	Rep	Wt	Rep	Wt	Rep	Wt	Rep	Wt	Rep

Introduction to Exercises

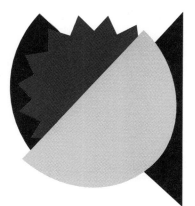

DIVISION OF EXERCISES

The weight training exercises presented in this book have been arranged into the following chapters.

Chapter 7 — Chest Exercises
Chapter 8 — Back Exercises (Lats and Traps)
Chapter 9 — Shoulder Exercises
Chapter 10 — Arm Exercises
Chapter 11 — Leg Exercises
Chapter 12 — Abdominal and Back Extension Exercises

The exercise descriptions in this book are consistent with the exercise technique recommendations of the National Strength and Conditioning Association (NSCA). The general pattern in these chapters is to present a basic barbell and dumbbell exercise on the left page along with a description of the exercise and an illustration of the major muscles used to perform the exercise. Then, on the right page directly across from it are common exercise machine positions for the same exercise. A variety of exercise machines have been used because there are many good ones on the market.

The idea is for you to recognize that you can either perform the basic barbell/dumbbell exercise or perform the same exercise movement on the machines you have available, and realize you are working the same muscles.

Some exercise machines use a cam or a pivot system to vary the resistance as you move through the range of motion. This is not really very important for you to understand as a beginner as long as you provide your muscles with an appropriate overload stimulus.

The *concentric phase* of a weight training exercise is the portion of the exercise during which the muscular contractions overcome the resistance and the weight is lifted. The *eccentric phase* of a weight training exercise is the portion of the exercise during which the resistance overcomes the muscular contraction and the weight is lowered. The same muscles are working during both the concentric phase and the eccentric phase of a weight training exercise. Don't perform half an exercise; the weight should be controlled and the muscles loaded all the way up and all the way down.

Almost any barbell exercise can be performed using dumbbells. In many dumbbell exercises the dumbbells may be moved together or in an alternating manner.

Major Muscles of the Human Body

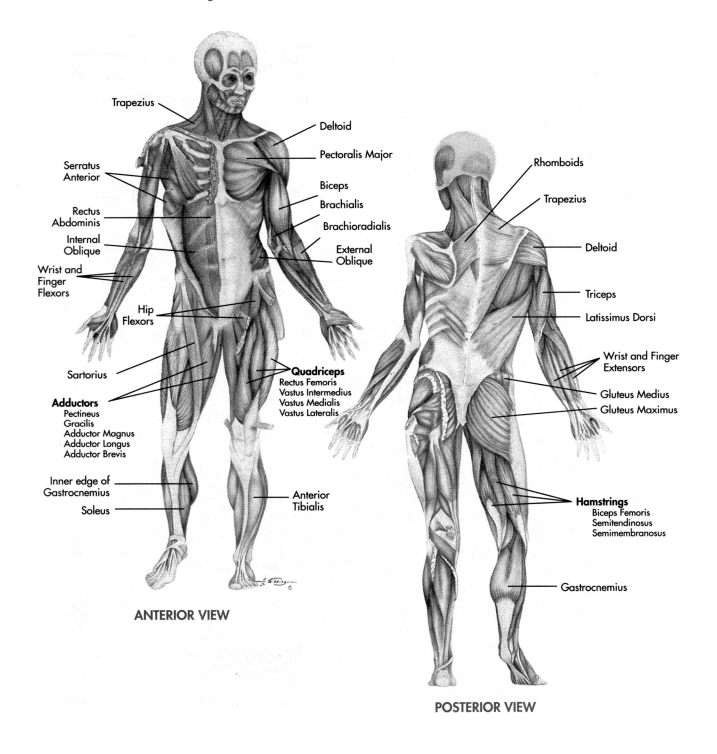

ANTERIOR VIEW

Trapezius

Deltoid

Pectoralis Major

Serratus Anterior

Biceps

Brachialis

Rectus Abdominis

Brachioradialis

Internal Oblique

External Oblique

Wrist and Finger Flexors

Hip Flexors

Sartorius

Quadriceps
Rectus Femoris
Vastus Intermedius
Vastus Medialis
Vastus Lateralis

Adductors
Pectineus
Gracilis
Adductor Magnus
Adductor Longus
Adductor Brevis

Inner edge of Gastrocnemius

Anterior Tibialis

Soleus

POSTERIOR VIEW

Rhomboids

Trapezius

Deltoid

Triceps

Latissimus Dorsi

Wrist and Finger Extensors

Gluteus Medius

Gluteus Maximus

Hamstrings
Biceps Femoris
Semitendinosus
Semimembranosus

Gastrocnemius

From *Basic Physiology and Anatomy* by E. Chaffee and F. Lytle (Philadelphia: Lippincott Co., 1980). Reproduced by permission.

Chest Exercises

7

◗ Chest (Pectoralis major)

- ◗ Barbell Bench Press
- ◗ Dumbbell Bench Press
- ◗ Universal Prone Bench Press Machine
- ◗ Cybex Seated Chest Press Machine

- ◗ Incline Barbell Bench Press
- ◗ Incline Dumbbell Bench Press
- ◗ Boss Incline Bench Press Machine
- ◗ Cybex Incline Bench Press Machine

- ◗ Bent-Arm Dumbbell Flyes
- ◗ Body Master Bent-Arm Machine Flyes
- ◗ Universal Chest Press or Pec Deck Machine
- ◗ Nautilus 10-Degree Chest Machine

◗ Chest/Back (Pectoralis major and Latissimus dorsi)

- ◗ Barbell Bent-Arm Pullover
- ◗ Dumbbell Straight-Arm Pullover
- ◗ Universal Bent-Arm Pullover Machine
- ◗ Nautilus Pullover Machine

CHEST

BENCH PRESS

Muscles developed: Pectoralis major, anterior deltoid, triceps.

Starting position: Start on your back on a flat bench; hold a barbell directly above your shoulders, arms straight, and both feet flat on the floor (A).

Eccentric phase: Inhale as you lower the bar to touch your chest (B).

Concentric phase: Exhale as you press the weight back up to the starting position.

Spotting: Have a spotter stand at the head end of the bench in case you cannot press the weight back to the starting position.

Variations: Change the angle of the bench and change the width of the hand spacing on the bar to achieve many variations of this basic chest exercise. You may also choose to perform this exercise with dumbbells.

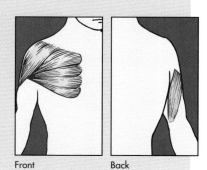

Front   Back

Additional information: To make this exercise easier to perform, use a rack to hold the weight above the bench. Some people prefer to place their feet on the bench to keep the lower back flat on the bench.

Caution: Do not arch your lower back during this lift.

Barbell

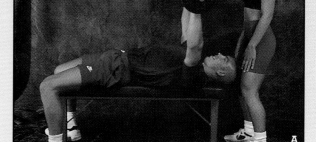

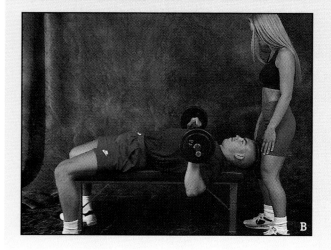

Dumbbell

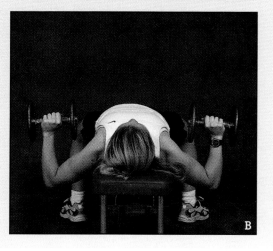

UNIVERSAL PRONE BENCH PRESS

Muscles developed:
Pectoralis major, anterior deltoid, triceps.

Starting position:
Start on your back on a flat bench; grasp the bar with your hands wider than shoulder width and your elbows bent; place both feet flat on the floor or on the end of the bench (A).

Concentric phase:
Exhale as you press the weight upward to a straight arm position (B).

Eccentric phase:
Inhale as you lower the weight to the starting position.

Cautions:

1. Do not arch your lower back or lift your hips off of the bench during the performance of this lift.

2. Keep your head a safe distance away from the weight stack and the selector pin.

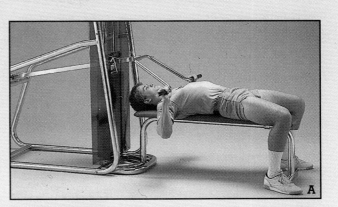

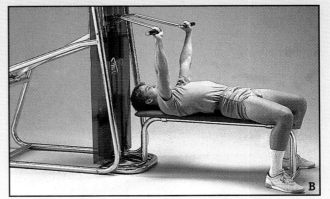

CYBEX SEATED CHEST PRESS

Muscles developed:
Pectoralis major, anterior deltoid, triceps.

Starting position:
Adjust the machine so you start in a seated position with the exercise handles at chest level. Grasp the exercise handles with your hands wider than shoulder width and your elbows bent (A).

Concentric phase:
Exhale as you press forward to a straight arm position (B).

Eccentric phase:
Inhale as you allow the weight to return to the starting position.

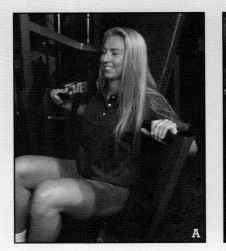

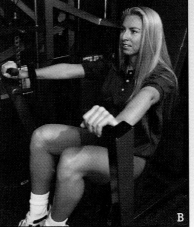

INCLINE BENCH PRESS

Muscles developed: Upper pectoralis major, anterior deltoid, triceps.

Starting position: Start on your back on an incline bench; hold a barbell directly above your shoulders with both arms straight, and both feet flat on the floor (A).

Eccentric phase: Inhale as you lower the bar to touch your chest (B).

Concentric phase: Exhale as you press the weight back up to the starting position.

Spotting: Have a spotter stand behind the bench in case you cannot get the weight back to the starting position.

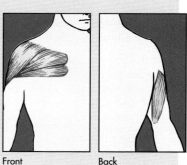

Front   Back

Variations:

1. Change the angle of the incline bench.
2. Change your hand spacing on the bar.
3. Use dumbbells instead of a barbell.

Additional Information:
To make this exercise easier to perform, use a weight rack to support the weight above the bench.

Barbell

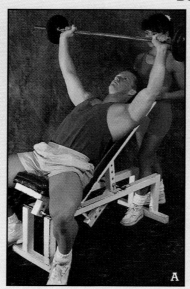
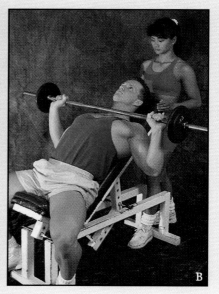

Dumbbell

Caution:
Dumbbells can be difficult to control because they are free to move in any direction. Begin with a light weight and master the movement before using heavier dumbbells. Have a spotter in position to help if you do begin to lose control of the exercise movement.

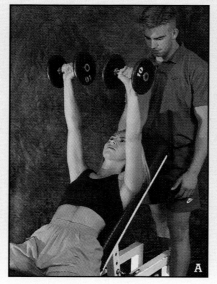
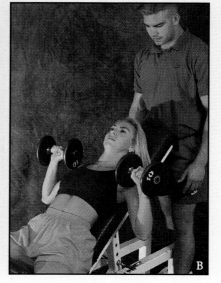

BOSS INCLINE BENCH PRESS

Muscles developed: Upper pectoralis major, anterior deltoid, triceps.

Starting position: Start in a seated position on an incline bench press machine (A).

Concentric phase: Exhale as you press the weight upward to a straight arm position (B).

Eccentric phase: Inhale as you slowly lower the weight to the starting position.

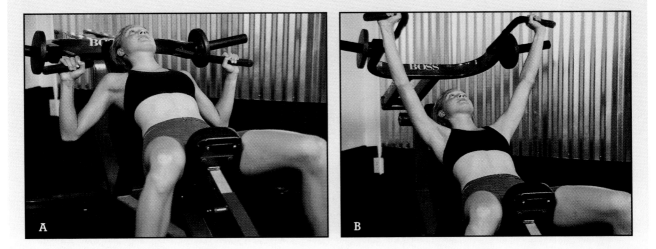

CYBEX INCLINE BENCH PRESS

Muscles developed:
Upper pectoralis major, anterior deltoid, triceps.

Starting position:
Start in a seated position on an incline bench press machine (A).

Concentric phase:
Exhale as you press the weight upward to a straight arm

position (B).

Eccentric phase:
Inhale as you slowly lower the weight to the starting position.

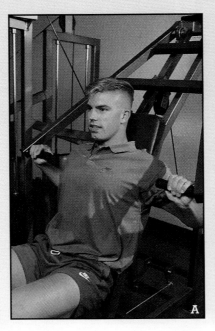
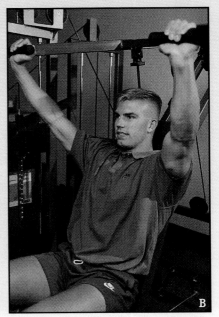

BENT-ARM FLYES

Muscles developed: Pectoralis major, anterior deltoid.

Starting position: Start on your back on a flat exercise bench; hold one dumbbell in each hand above your shoulders, with your arms slightly bent (A).

Eccentric phase: Inhale as you move the dumbbells away from each other and lower them toward the floor (B).

Concentric phase: Exhale as you return the dumbbells to the starting position.

Variations: Perform this exercise on an incline or decline bench.

Additional information: Keep your elbows slightly bent throughout this exercise to place the exercise stress on the pectoralis major muscle and relieve the stress on the elbow joint.

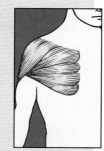

Front

Dumbbell

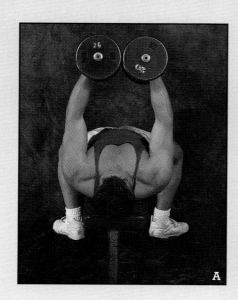

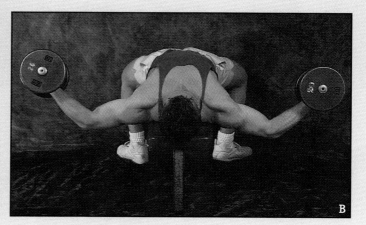

A

B

Body Master Machine

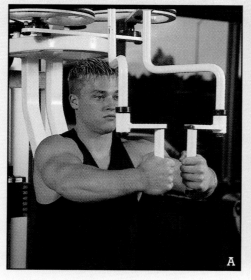

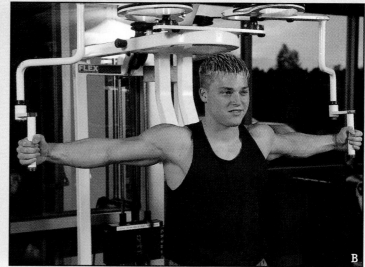

A

B

UNIVERSAL CHEST PRESS OR PEC DECK

Muscles developed:
Pectoralis major, anterior deltoid.

Starting position:
Start in a seated position with your elbows bent and your forearms on the padded exercise bars. Adjust the seat so that your elbows are shoulder height (A).

Concentric phase:
Exhale as you pull your arms forward and toward each other. Keep pulling until the exercise bars gently touch each other (B).

Eccentric phase:
Inhale as you slowly allow your arms to return to the starting position.

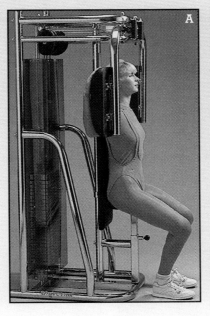
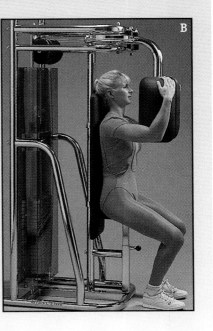

NAUTILUS 10-DEGREE CHEST MACHINE

Muscles developed:
Pectoralis major, anterior deltoid.

Starting position:
Start on your back on the bench and place your arms under the padded exercise bars. (see photo)

Concentric phase:
Exhale as you pull your bent arms upward and toward each other. Keep pulling until the exercise bars gently touch each other or come to the end of their travel. Pause briefly and try to squeeze your arms together.

Eccentric phase:
Inhale as you slowly allow your arms to return to the starting position.

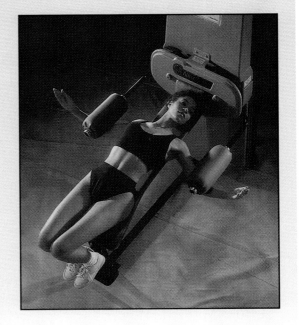

CHEST / BACK

BARBELL BENT-ARM PULLOVER

Muscles developed: Latissimus dorsi, pectoralis major.

Starting position: Start on your back on a flat bench; hold a barbell supported on your chest, hands 6 to 12 inches apart, elbows bent, and head beyond the end of the bench (A).

Eccentric phase: Inhale as you lower the weight past your face toward the floor (B).

Concentric phase: Exhale as you pull the weight back to the starting position.

Additional information: Keep your elbows bent and your arms in close to your head.

Caution: Keep your arms pressed inward toward your head to avoid placing too much strain on the medial side of your elbow joints.

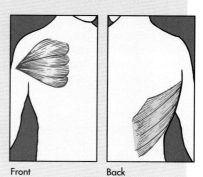

Front   Back

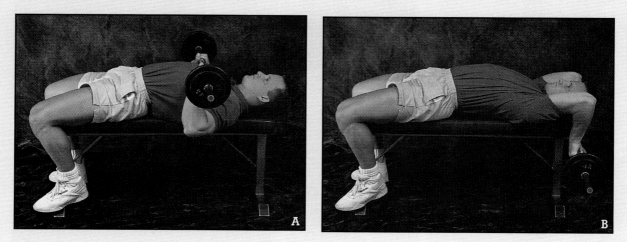

DUMBBELL STRAIGHT-ARM PULLOVER

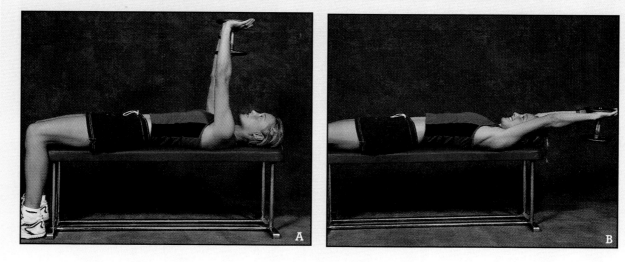

UNIVERSAL BENT-ARM PULLOVER

Muscles developed:
Pectoralis major, Latissimus dorsi.

Starting position:
Start in a seated position with your shoulder joints aligned with the pivot point of the machine. Fasten the seat belt to hold your hips in the correct position. Grasp the exercise bar behind your head with a palms-up grip (A).

Concentric phase:
Exhale as you pull the exercise bar over your head and all the way to your abdomen (B).

Eccentric phase:
Inhale as you slowly allow the bar to return to the starting position.

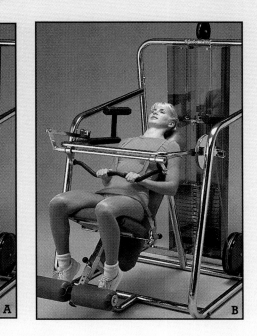

Caution:
Keep your arms in close to your head to avoid strain on the medial side of your elbow joints.

NAUTILUS PULLOVER

Muscles developed:
Pectoralis major, Latissimus dorsi.

Starting position:
Start in a seated position with your shoulder joints aligned with the pivot point of the pullover machine. Fasten the seat belt to hold your hips in the correct position. Push down on the foot bar to bring the exercise bar forward to a position where you can place your upper arms on the padded portion of the exercise bar as shown in the photograph (A). Allow the bar to gently pull your arms back to the starting position, then remove your feet from the foot bar.

Concentric phase:
Exhale as you pull the exercise bar over your head and all the way to your abdomen (B).

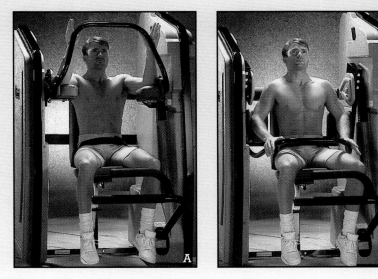

Eccentric phase: Inhale as you slowly allow the exercise bar to return to the starting position.

Back Exercises

🔖 Back (Latissimus dorsi)

- 🔖 Barbell Rowing
- 🔖 One-Dumbbell Rowing
- 🔖 Cybex Seated Rowing Machine
- 🔖 Nautilus Seated Rowing Machine

- 🔖 Pull-Ups
- 🔖 Chin-Ups
- 🔖 Universal Lat Pulldown
- 🔖 Cybex Weight-Assisted Pull-Up

🔖 Upper Back (Trapezius)

- 🔖 Barbell Shoulder Shrug
- 🔖 Dumbbell Shoulder Shrug
- 🔖 Low Pulley Shoulder Shrug
- 🔖 Nautilus Shoulder Shrug Machine

BACK (Lats)

ROWING

Muscles developed: Latissimus dorsi, teres major, posterior deltoid, trapezius, rhomboids.

Starting position: Bend over with your knees slightly bent; hold a barbell in your hands with your arms straight so that the barbell is hanging directly below your shoulders (A).

Concentric phase: Exhale as the weight is pulled upward (B) until the bar touches your chest. Pause briefly with the bar held against your chest.

Eccentric phase: Inhale as the weight is lowered slowly to the starting position.

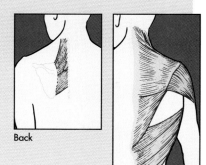

Back

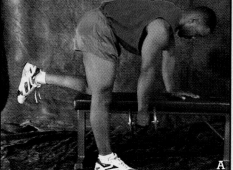

Back

Variations:

1. Stand on a bench or block to get more stretch in the starting position as the weight increases and larger plates are used.

2. Change the distance between your hands.

3. Pull the bar to your shoulders or chest, or abdomen.

4. Perform this exercise with dumbbells, bringing both up at the same time or alternately.

Additional information:
Keep your back flat throughout this exercise. Do not jerk or drop the weight. Keep your knees bent slightly to reduce the stress on your lower back.

Caution:
Your lower back will be in a potentially dangerous position. To make this exercise safer for your lower back, perform it with your forehead supported lightly on a solid object that is about waist high.

Barbell

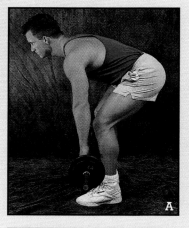

A

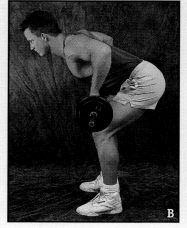

B

One-Dumbbell

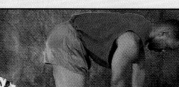

A

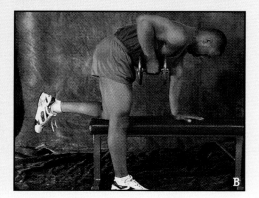

B

CYBEX SEATED ROWING

Muscles developed: Latissimus dorsi, teres major, posterior deltoid, trapezius, rhomboids.

Starting position: Adjust the chest pad so you can just reach the handles of the exercise bar with your arms fully extended (A).

Concentric phase: Exhale as you pull the exercise handles toward your chest (B). Pause briefly in the fully contracted position.

Eccentric phase: Inhale as you slowly allow the exercise handles to return to the starting position.

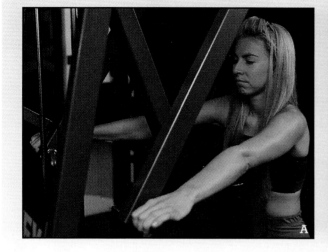

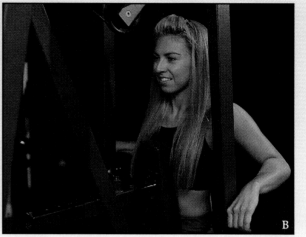

NAUTILUS SEATED ROWING

Muscles developed: Latissimus dorsi, teres major, posterior deltoid, trapezius, rhomboids.

Starting position: Start facing the machine and grasp one exercise bar in each hand.

Concentric phase: Exhale as you pull the exercise bars toward your chest. Pause briefly in the fully contracted position and squeeze your shoulder blades together.

Eccentric phase: Inhale as you slowly allow the exercise bars to return to the starting position.

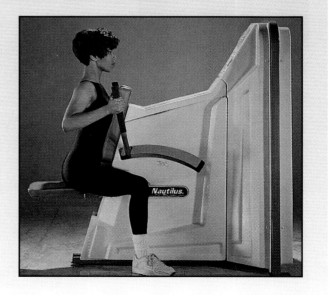

PULL-UPS

Muscles developed: Latissimus dorsi, teres major, biceps brachii.

Starting position: Hang from a bar with a pronated (thumbs in) grip (A).

Concentric phase: Exhale as you pull yourself upward to a position with your chin above the bar (B).

Eccentric phase: Inhale as you lower yourself slowly to the starting position.

Variations: Change grip direction and spacing for several good variations of this exercise.

Additional information: Start each pull-up from a full hang. Pause with your chin above the bar, and lower yourself slowly to the starting position. Add weight by suspending a dumbbell from a wide strap that passes around your lower back and placing the dumbbell between your thighs.

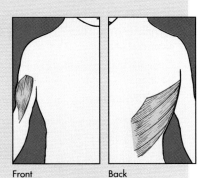

Front   Back

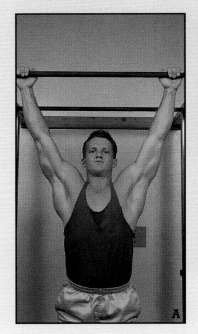

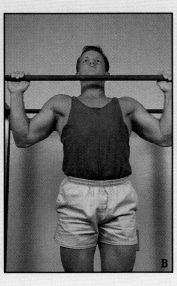

CHIN-UPS

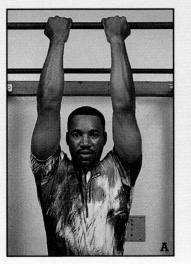

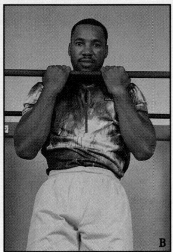

UNIVERSAL LAT PULLDOWN

Muscles developed:
Latissimus dorsi, teres major, biceps.

Starting position:
Grasp the bar with a pronated grip and your hands wider than shoulder width. Assume a seated position with your arms straight (A).

Concentric phase:
Inhale and pull the exercise bar down to your upper chest (B). Pause briefly in the fully contracted position and squeeze your shoulder blades together.

Eccentric phase:
Exhale as you slowly allow the exercise bar to return to the starting position.

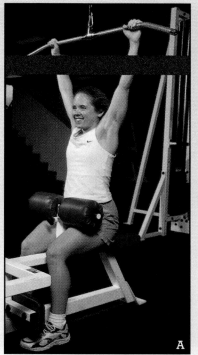
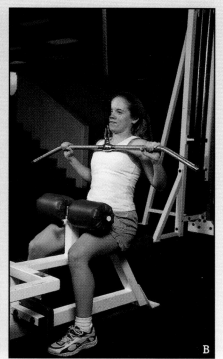

CYBEX WEIGHT-ASSISTED PULL-UP

Muscles developed:
Latissimus dorsi, teres major, biceps.

Starting position:
Set the weight for the amount of assistance you want from the machine. Grasp the overhead bar with a pronated grip. Step from the platform onto the weight-assist bar and lower yourself to the fully stretched starting position (A).

Concentric phase:
Exhale as you pull yourself upward to a position with your chin above the bar (B). Pause briefly and squeeze your shoulder blades together.

Eccentric phase:
Inhale as you lower yourself slowly to the starting position.

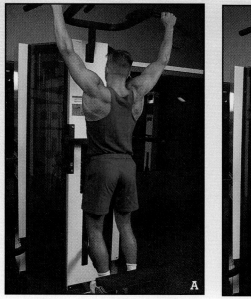
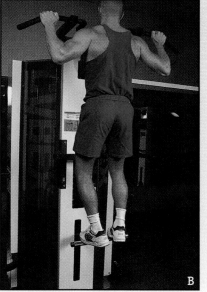

UPPER BACK (Traps)

SHOULDER SHRUG

Muscles developed: Trapezius, levator scapulae.

Starting position: Start with a barbell hanging at arms length in front of your body; hold the bar with both hands in a pronated (thumbs in) grip (A).

Concentric phase: Inhale as you lift or shrug your shoulders to the highest possible position (B). Hold that position briefly.

Eccentric phase: Exhale as you slowly lower the bar to the starting position.

Variations:

1. Roll your shoulders forward and up, then back and down.
2. Roll your shoulders back and up, then forward and down.

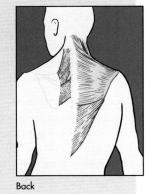

Back

Barbell

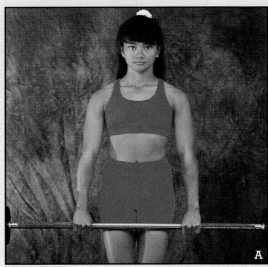

A

Additional information: Do not bend your elbows or pull with your arm muscles. The hands and arms serve as hooks to hang the weight on during this exercise. Do not jerk the weight upward or let it drop back to the starting position.

Dumbbell

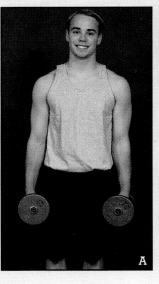

A

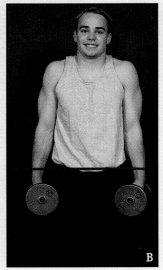

B

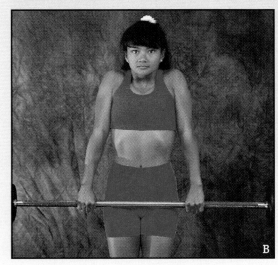

B

LOW PULLEY SHOULDER SHRUG

Muscles developed:
Trapezius, levator scapulae.

Starting position:
Start in a standing position holding
the low pulley handle with a pronated
grip. With your arms straight, allow the
weight to pull your shoulders down as
far as possible (A).

Concentric phase:
Inhale as you pull your shoulders
upward as high as possible while
keeping your arms straight (B).
Pause briefly and hold this position.

Eccentric phase:
Exhale as you slowly lower the
weight to the starting position.

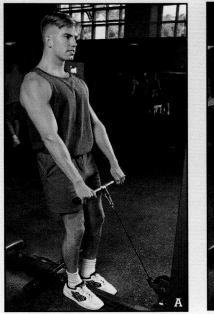
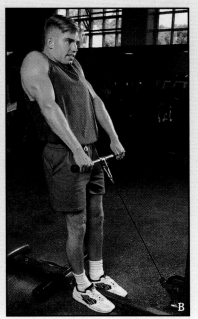

NAUTILUS SHOULDER SHRUG

Muscles developed: Trapezius, levator scapulae.

Starting position: Start in a seated position with your
forearms between the padded exercise bars.

Concentric phase: Inhale as you pull your shoulders upward
as high as possible. Pause briefly at the top of the pull and hold
this position.

Eccentric phase: Exhale as you slowly lower the weight to the
starting position.

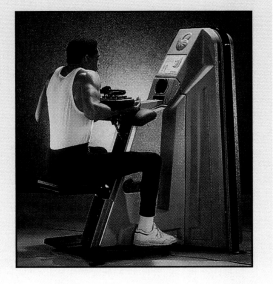

Shoulder Exercises

🔹 Shoulder (Deltoid)

- 🔹 Barbell Overhead Press or Military Press
- 🔹 Dumbbell Overhead Press
- 🔹 Hammer Strength Overhead Press Machine
- 🔹 Boss Overhead Press Machine

- 🔹 Barbell Upright Rowing
- 🔹 Dumbbell Upright Rowing
- 🔹 Universal Low Pulley Upright Rowing (Separate Handles)
- 🔹 Low Pulley Upright Rowing (Straight Bar)

- 🔹 Dumbbell Lateral Raise
- 🔹 Cybex Seated Lateral Raise Machine
- 🔹 Dumbbell Front Raise
- 🔹 Dumbbell Bent-Over Lateral Raise

OVERHEAD PRESS OR MILITARY PRESS

Muscles developed: Deltoid, triceps.

Starting position: Start with a barbell supported at shoulder level in front of your body, your hands placed slightly wider apart than shoulder-width (A).

Concentric phase: Inhale while pressing the weight overhead to a straight arm position (B).

Eccentric phase: Exhale while lowering the weight to the starting position.

Variations: There are many variations of this overhead press. It can be done standing or sitting, with a barbell from the shoulders in front of the head or behind the neck, with dumbbells together or alternating.

Caution: Do **not** lean back or arch your back. Do not close your eyes.

Additional information: This exercise is called the military press because you stay in an erect posture (military posture) while forcing the muscles of the arms and shoulders to do all the work. Do not bend or sway the back to complete a repetition.

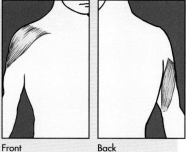

Front   Back

Barbell

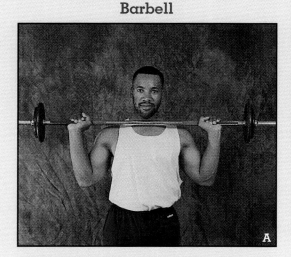

A

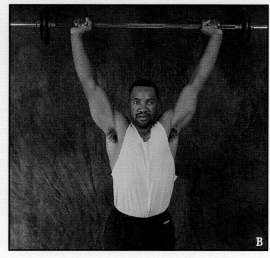

B

Dumbbell

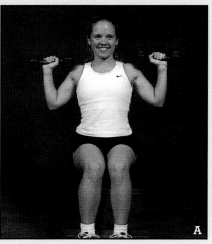

A

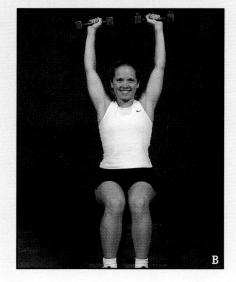

B

HAMMER STRENGTH OVERHEAD PRESS

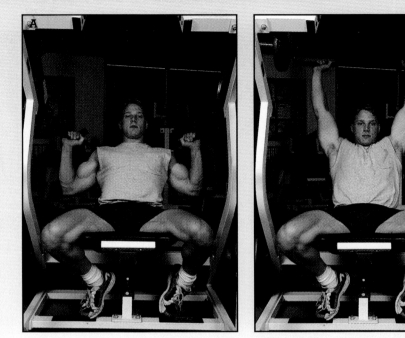

Muscles developed:
Deltoid, triceps.

Starting position:
Start in a seated position. Grasp the exercise bars with your hands wider than shoulder width (A).

Concentric phase:
Inhale as you press the exercise bar upward to a straight arm position (B).

Eccentric phase:
Exhale as you slowly lower the weight to the starting position.

BOSS OVERHEAD PRESS MACHINE

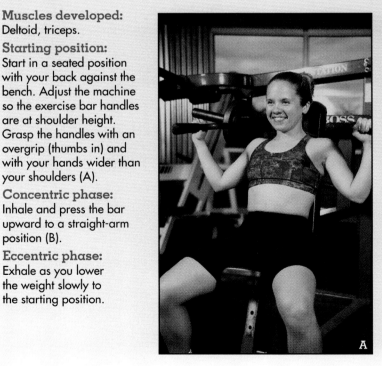
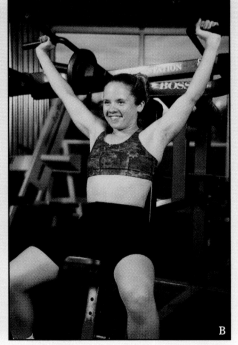

Muscles developed:
Deltoid, triceps.

Starting position:
Start in a seated position with your back against the bench. Adjust the machine so the exercise bar handles are at shoulder height. Grasp the handles with an overgrip (thumbs in) and with your hands wider than your shoulders (A).

Concentric phase:
Inhale and press the bar upward to a straight-arm position (B).

Eccentric phase:
Exhale as you lower the weight slowly to the starting position.

UPRIGHT ROWING

Muscles developed: Deltoid, trapezius.

Starting position: Start with a barbell hanging at arm's length in front of your body, hands in a pronated (thumbs in) grip (A).

Concentric phase: Inhale while pulling the elbows as high as possible in a smooth, continuous movement. The bar should reach shoulder level (B).

Eccentric phase: Exhale while lowering the bar slowly to the starting position.

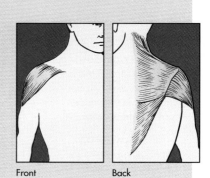

Front   Back

Additional information: Concentrate on your deltoid muscles while raising the upper arm and keeping your elbows high. The arm muscles should be as inactive as possible. Upright rowing is like performing lateral raises, but with a barbell instead of dumbbells.

Barbell

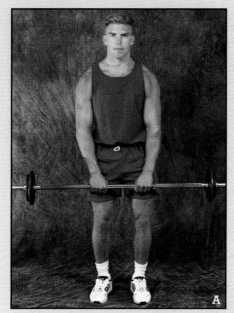

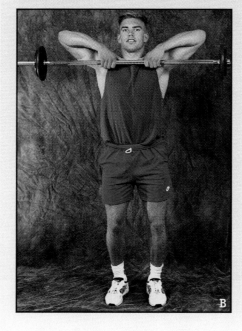

Dumbbell

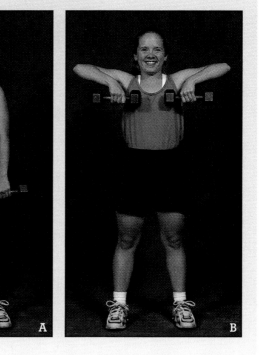

UNIVERSAL LOW PULLEY UPRIGHT ROWING
(Separate Handles)

Muscles developed:
Deltoid, trapezius.

Starting position:
Start in a standing position facing the low pulley station. Hold the exercise handle or handles on the end of the cable (A).

Concentric phase:
Inhale as you pull your elbows upward as high as possible in a smooth, continuous movement. Pull your elbows upward until your hands reach shoulder or chin height (B).

Eccentric phase:
Exhale as you lower the weight slowly to the starting position.

Additional information:
Your elbows always should be higher than your hands during this exercise.

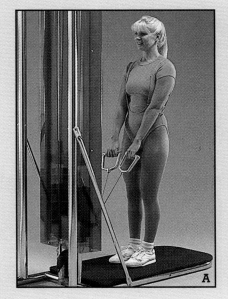
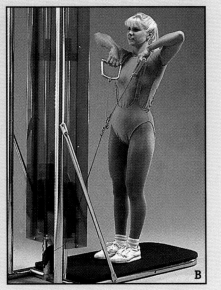

LOW PULLEY UPRIGHT ROWING
(Straight Bar)

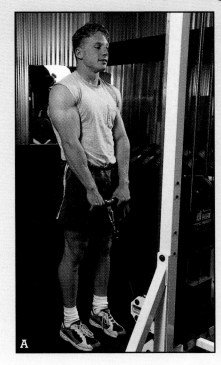
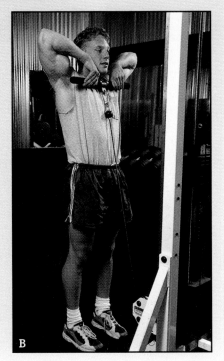

DUMBBELL LATERAL RAISE

Muscles developed: Deltoid, trapezius.

Starting position: Start with one dumbbell in each hand (A).

Concentric phase: Inhale while lifting the weights away from your body and upward. Keep your arms fairly straight, and raise the weights to shoulder level (B).

Eccentric phase: Exhale while lowering the weights to the starting position.

Variations: Perform the same exercise movement from a sitting position. The deltoid is a muscle with three fairly distinct parts: anterior (front), lateral (middle), and posterior (rear). The lateral raise tends to best develop the lateral part; the front raise develops the front part; and the bent-over lateral raise develops the rear part.

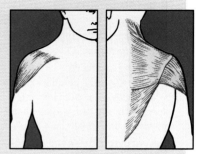

Front   Back

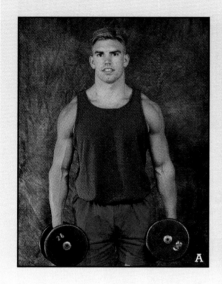

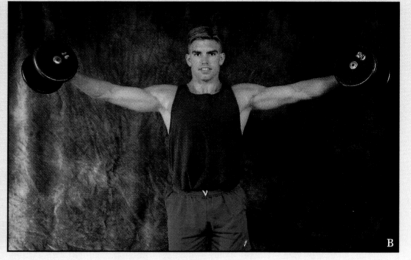

CYBEX SEATED LATERAL RAISE

Muscles developed: Deltoid, trapezius.

Starting position: Start in a seated position. Adjust the machine so your shoulders are lined up with the pivot points of the machine. Place your arms against the padded portion of the exercise bars (A).

Concentric phase: Inhale as you press your upper arms outward and upward to a position in which your elbows are shoulder height or slightly above (B). Pause briefly at the top.

Eccentric phase: Exhale as you slowly allow your arms to return to the starting position.

Additional Information: To focus more on the lateral part of the deltoid, keep your forearms pointing forward. To focus more on the frontal part of the deltoid, have your forearms pointing outward and upward.

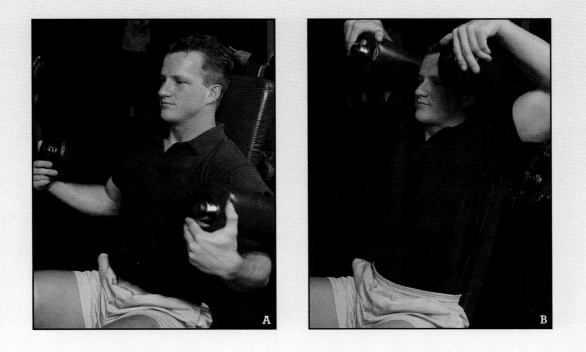

DUMBBELL FRONT RAISE

Muscles developed: Frontal deltoid, clavicular portion of pectoralis major, coracobrachialis.

Starting position: Stand and hold a barbell or two dumbbells at arms length (A).

Concentric phase: Inhale while raising the weight to shoulder level, keeping your arms straight (B). Pause briefly.

Eccentric phase: Exhale while lowering the weight to the starting position.

Variations: Raise the weight to an overhead position, as long as you do not allow your back to arch or bend.

Note: On straight-arm exercises a slight bend at the elbow may relieve unnecessary tension or strain in the elbow joint. This is not a problem as long as it makes the exercise more productive for you. But do not bend your elbows to make the exercise easier for the working muscles.

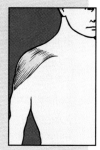

Front

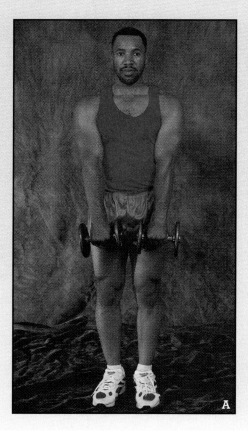

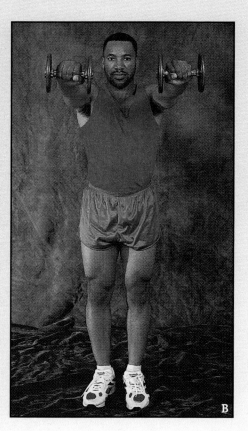

DUMBBELL BENT-OVER LATERAL RAISE

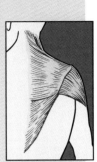

Back

Muscles developed: Posterior (rear) deltoid, rhomboids, trapezius.

Starting position: Bend over with your back flat and knees slightly bent; hold one dumbbell in each hand, arms straight, and dumbbells hanging directly below your shoulder joints (A).

Concentric phase: Inhale while raising the dumbbells to the side up to shoulder level (B). Pause briefly.

Eccentric phase: Exhale while lowering the weights slowly to the starting position.

Variations: Sit on the end of a bench or lie face down on a flat or incline bench that is high enough to allow your arms to hang fully extended.

Additional information: Lift your arms straight to the side or move them slightly forward toward your head as the weight is lifted. These muscles also are developed when performing any of the rowing exercises for the back (lats).

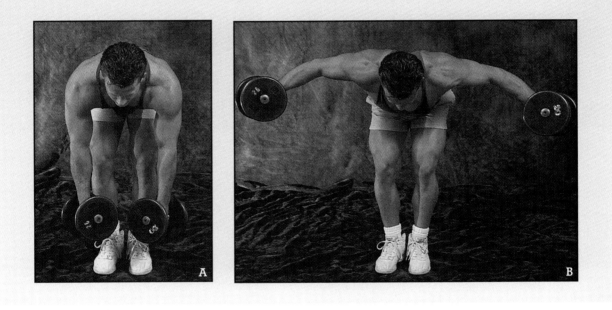

Arm Exercises

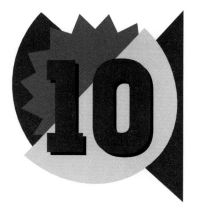

Upper Arm (Elbow flexion, Biceps)

- Barbell Curl
- Dumbbell Curl
- Universal Arm Curl Machine
- Nautilus Arm Curl Machine

- Barbell Reverse Curl
- Incline Dumbbell Curl
- Hammer Strength Arm Curl Machine
- Low Pulley Curl

Upper Arm (Elbow extension, Triceps)

- Barbell Triceps Extension
- One-Dumbbell Triceps Extension
- Nautilus Triceps Extension Machine
- Universal Triceps Pushdown

- Parallel Bar Dips
- Bench Dips
- Boss Dip Machine
- Cybex Weight-Assisted Parallel Bar Dips

- Lying Barbell Triceps Extension
- Close-Grip Bench Press
- Body Master Triceps Extension
- Close-Grip Bench Press on Smith Machine

Forearm (Wrist flexors and Wrist extensors)

- Barbell Wrist Curl
- Dumbbell Wrist Curl
- Reverse Barbell Wrist Curl
- Reverse Dumbbell Wrist Curl

UPPER ARM (Elbow Flexion)

BARBELL CURL

Muscles developed: Biceps brachii, brachialis, brachioradialis.

Starting position: Stand, holding a barbell in front of your body, hands gripping the bar at shoulder width with a supinated (thumbs out) grip (A).

Concentric phase: Exhale while raising the weight to your shoulders by moving only at the elbow joint (B).

Eccentric phase: Inhale while lowering the weight to the starting position.

Variations: Any elbow flexion or curling exercise will develop the elbow flexor muscles. Curling exercises have many variations. Vary this standing curl by changing the space between your hands when gripping the bar.

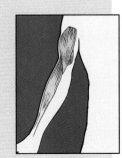

Front

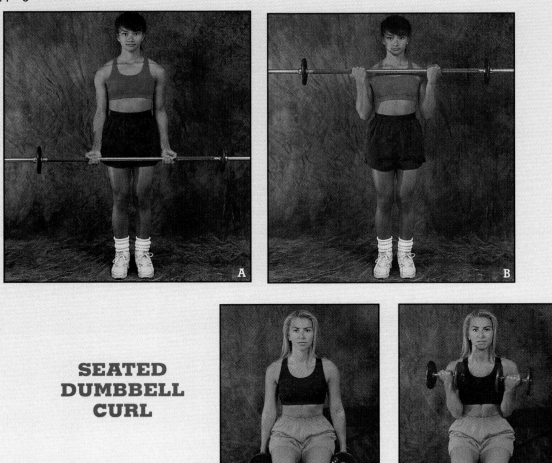

SEATED DUMBBELL CURL

UNIVERSAL ARM CURL

Muscles developed:
Biceps, brachialis, brachioradialis.

Starting position:
Start in a seated position. Grasp the exercise handles and line your elbow joints up with the pivot point of the exercise machine (A). Straighten your arms.

Concentric phase:
Exhale as you pull upward on the exercise handles, moving only your hands and forearms (B). Continue pulling until your hands are near your shoulders and your forearms will not move any closer to your upper arm.

Eccentric phase:
Inhale as you lower the weight slowly to the starting position with your arms fully extended.

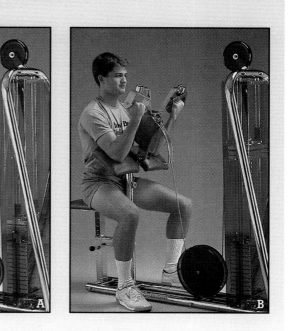

Caution:
Do **not** hyperextend your elbows or allow the weight to overstretch the elbow joints at the bottom of the eccentric phase.

NAUTILUS ARM CURL MACHINE

Muscles developed:
Biceps, brachialis, brachioradialis.

Starting position:
Grasp the exercise handles of the machine with a palms-up grip; place your elbows on the pad, and line them up with the pivot point of the machine (A).

Concentric phase:
Exhale as you pull your hands toward your shoulders (B). When you reach the end of your elbow joint range of motion, pause briefly and hold.

Eccentric phase:
Inhale as you lower the weight slowly and allow your arms to return to the starting position.

Caution:
Do **not** jerk the weight up or allow

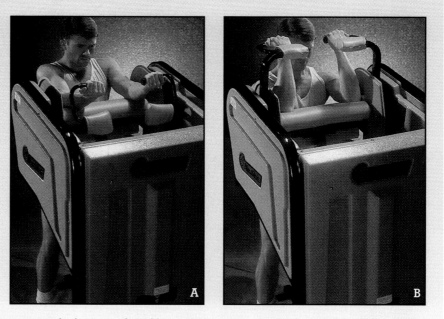

it to drop and hyperextend your elbow joints at the bottom. Lift and lower the weight in a smooth and controlled manner.

BARBELL REVERSE CURL

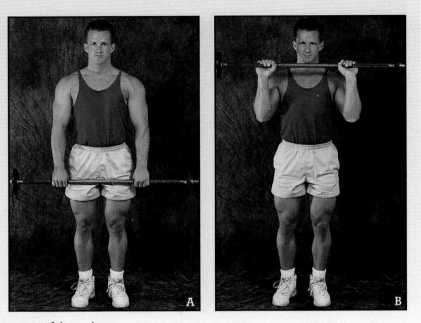

Muscles developed:
Biceps, brachialis, brachioradialis, wrist and hand flexors.

Starting position:
Stand and hold a barbell in front of your body with both hands in a pronated (thumbs in) grip (A).

Concentric phase:
Exhale while raising the bar to the shoulders by bending only at the elbows (B).

Eccentric phase:
Inhale while lowering the bar to the starting position.

Variations:
Change the distance between your hands.

Additional information:
This exercise provides a strong stimulus to the forearm muscles and often is used as a forearm exercise as well as a variation of the curl.

INCLINE DUMBBELL CURL

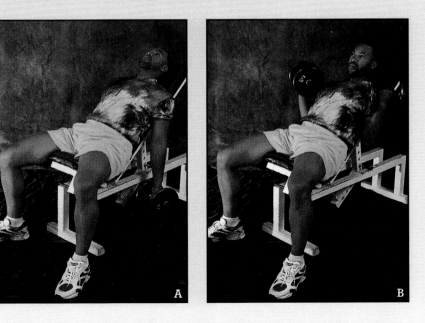

Muscles developed:
Biceps brachii, brachialis, brachiordialis.

Starting Position:
With your back against an incline bench, hold one dumbbell in each hand with your arms extended and hanging directly below your shoulder joints (A).

Concentric phase:
Exhale while bending your arms only at the elbow. Pull the weights to your shoulders (B).

Eccentric phase:
Inhale while lowering weights to the starting position.

Variations:
1. Alternate arms so that one is coming up as the other is going down.
2. Turn your arms out so the dumbbells are raised and lowered to the sides of your body instead of in front of your body.

HAMMER STRENGTH ARM CURL MACHINE

Muscles developed:
Biceps, brachialis, brachioradialis.

Starting position:
Grasp the exercise handles of the machine with a palms-up grip; place your elbows on the pad, and line them up with the pivot point of the machine (A).

Concentric phase:
Exhale as you pull your hands toward your shoulders (B). When you reach the end of your elbow joint range of motion, pause briefly and hold.

Eccentric phase:
Inhale as you lower the weight slowly and allow your arms to return to the starting position.

Caution:
Do **not** jerk the weight up or allow it to drop and hyperextend your elbow joints at the bottom. Lift and lower the weight in a smooth and controlled manner.

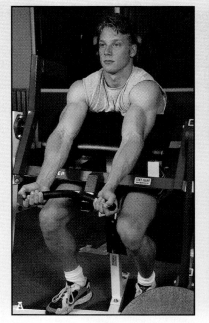
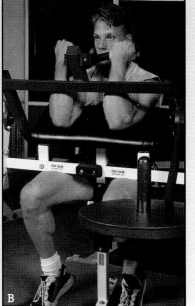

LOW PULLEY CURL

Muscles developed:
Biceps brachii, brachialis, brachioradialis.

Starting position:
Stand in front of the low pulley, facing the weight stack. Hold the exercise bar in a supinated (thumbs out) grip, with both arms straight (A).

Concentric phase:
Exhale as you bend only at the elbow joint to bring the exercise bar up toward your shoulders. Move only your forearms; do not allow your upper arms to change position (B).

Eccentric phase:
Inhale as you slowly lower the bar to the starting position.

Variations:
1. Change your grip spacing on the bar.
2. Use a pronated (thumbs in) grip and perform reverse curls.

Additional information:
You can cheat on this exercise in a number of ways. Bending any joint except the elbow joint will reduce the effectiveness of the exercise.

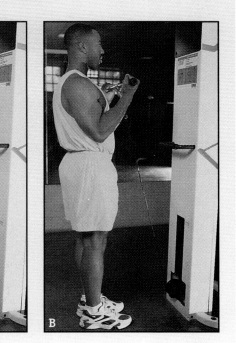

UPPER ARM (Elbow Extension)

TRICEPS EXTENSION

Muscles developed: Triceps.

Starting position: Stand and hold a barbell or dumbbell overhead with both hands (A).

Eccentric phase: Inhale as you slowly lower the weight behind your head (B).

Concentric phase: Exhale as you extend both arms and push the weight back to the starting position.

Variations:

1. Perform this exercise with a dumbbell.
2. Perform this exercise from a sitting position.

Additional information: Keep your elbows up throughout the exercise.

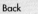

Back

Barbell

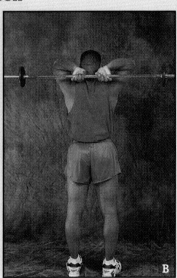
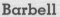

One-Dumbbell

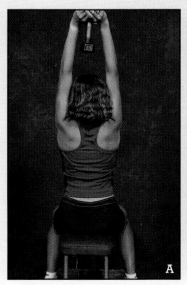
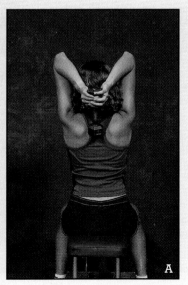

NAUTILUS TRICEPS EXTENSION MACHINE

Muscles developed:
Triceps.

Starting position:
Place the little finger side of your hands or fists against the padded portion of the exercise bars. With your elbows bent place the back of your upper arms on the pad provided and line up your elbow joints with the pivot point of the machine (A).

Concentric phase:
Exhale as you push both hands forward and downward until your arms are extended. Pause briefly and hold.

Eccentric phase:
Inhale as you allow your arms to slowly return to the starting position.

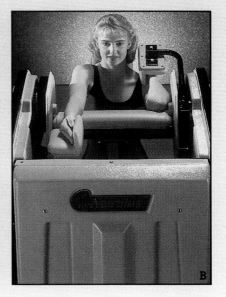

Variations:
This exercise also may be performed one arm at a time or alternating arms (B).

Caution:
Do **not** allow the weight to drop during the eccentric phase of the lift. Control the speed of the movement at all times.

UNIVERSAL TRICEPS PUSHDOWN

Muscles developed:
Triceps.

Starting position:
Place both hands on the high pulley bar (lat machine) with your palms down and your thumbs in (A).

Concentric phase:
Exhale as you push the bar down until your arms are straight (B). Throughout the exercise movement keep your upper arms by your sides and move only your hands and forearms.

Eccentric phase:
Inhale as you allow your hands and forearms to slowly return to the starting position.

Caution:
Keep your head, neck, and chest away from the moving cable.

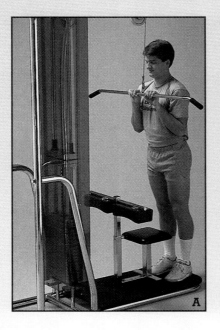

PARALLEL BAR DIPS

Muscles developed: Triceps, pectoralis major, anterior deltoid.

Starting position: Take a straight-arm support position on two bars parallel to each other and about shoulder width apart (A).

Eccentric phase: Inhale as you bend your elbows and slowly lower yourself as far as possible (B).

Concentric phase: Exhale as you straighten your arms and return to the starting position.

Additional information: To add weight to this exercise, hang a weight or a dumbbell from a wide strap around your waist and place it between your thighs to stabilize it during the exercise.

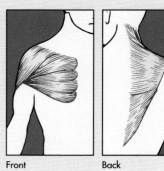

Front   Back

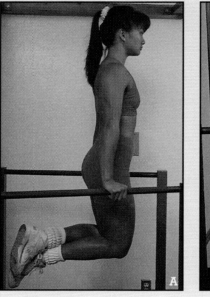

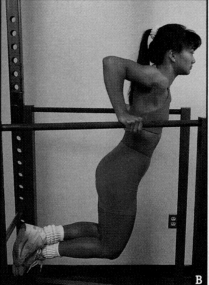

BENCH DIPS

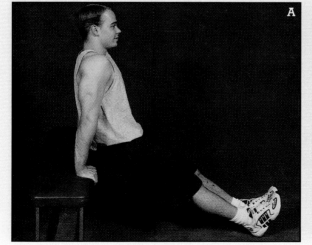

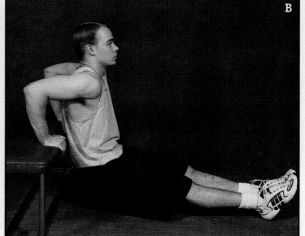

BOSS DIP MACHINE

Muscles developed:
Triceps, pectoralis major, anterior deltoid.

Starting position:
Start with your hands on the exercise bars (A).

Concentric phase:
Exhale as you press the exercise bar down until your arms are straight (B).

Eccentric phase:
Inhale as you slowly bend your arms and allow the weight to return to the starting position.

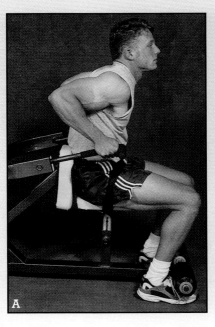
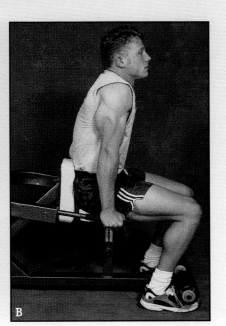

CYBEX WEIGHT-ASSISTED PARALLEL BAR DIPS

Muscles developed:
Triceps, pectoralis major, anterior deltoid.

Starting position:
Select the amount of weight assistance you want from the machine. Place your hands on the parallel bars, step from the platform onto the weight assist bar, and straighten your arms (A).

Eccentric phase:
Inhale as you bend your elbows and slowly lower yourself as far as possible (B).

Concentric phase:
Exhale as you straighten your arms and return to the starting position.

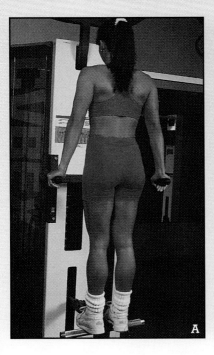
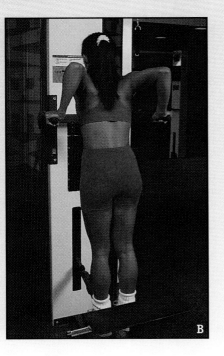

LYING BARBELL TRICEPS EXTENSION

Muscles developed:
Triceps.

Starting positions:
Start on your back on a flat exercise bench and hold a barbell above your shoulders, with both arms straight and your hands 6" to 8" apart (A).

Eccentric phase:
Inhale while lowering the bar to the top of your head by bending only at your elbows (B).

Concentric phase:
Exhale as you push the bar back to the starting position.

Variations:
Perform this exercise on an incline bench or a decline bench. Use one or two dumbbells in several variations.

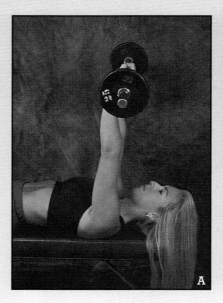
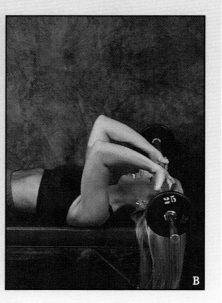

CLOSE-GRIP BENCH PRESS

Muscles developed:
Triceps, anterior deltoid, pectoralis major.

Starting position:
Start on your back on a flat bench and hold a barbell directly above your shoulders, with your arms straight and a close grip (hands 6" to 8" apart) (A).

Eccentric phase:
Inhale as you lower the bar until it touches your chest (B).

Concentric phase:
Exhale as you press the weight back to the starting position.

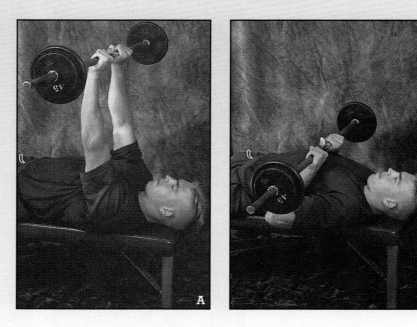

BODY MASTER TRICEPS EXTENSION

Muscles developed: Triceps.

Starting position: Sit on the triceps extension machine and grasp the bar with both elbows pointing up.

Eccentric phase: Inhale as you slowly lower the bar behind your head to the starting position.

Concentric phase: Exhale as you extend both arms and push the bar upward to a straight arm position.

Additional information: Keep your elbows pointing up throughout the exercise.

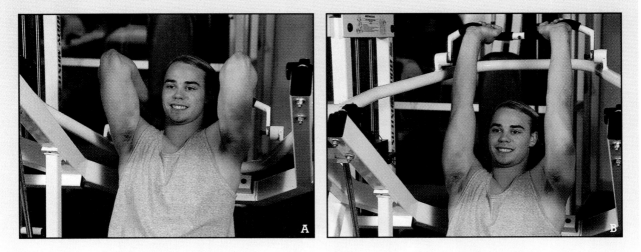

CLOSE-GRIP BENCH PRESS SMITH MACHINE

Muscles developed: Triceps, anterior deltoid, pectoralis major.

Starting position: Start on your back on a flat bench and hold a barbell directly above your shoulders, with your arms straight and a close grip (hands 6" to 8" apart) (A).

Eccentric phase: Inhale as you lower the bar until it touches your chest (B).

Concentric phase: Exhale as you press the weight back to the starting position.

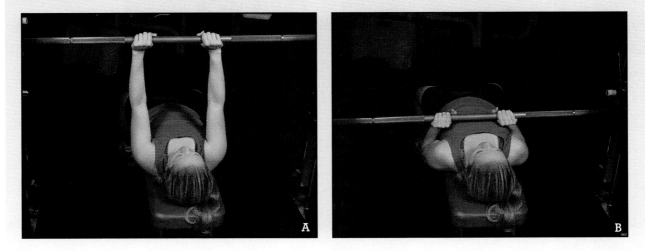

FOREARM

WRIST CURL

Muscles developed: Wrist and hand flexors.

Starting positions: Sit on an exercise bench and place your forearms on the bench with your wrists just beyond the end of the bench; hold a barbell with a supinated (thumbs out) grip, and allow the bar to hang toward the floor (A).

Concentric phase: Lift the weight, moving only your hands and wrists (B).

Eccentric phase: Lower the bar slowly to the starting position.

Variations: 1. Use one dumbbell in each hand.
2. Use one dumbbell and exercise one arm at a time.

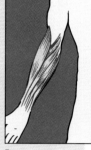

Front

Barbell

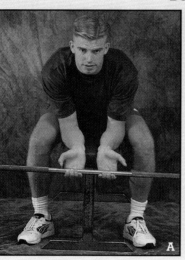
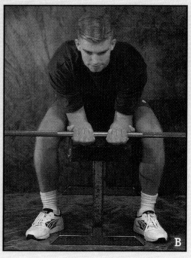

Dumbbell

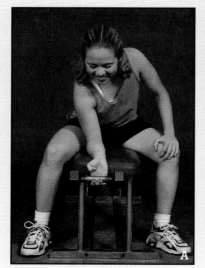
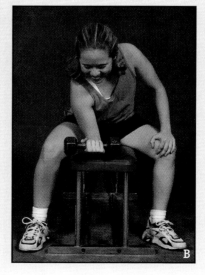

REVERSE WRIST CURL

Muscles developed: Wrist extensors.

Starting position: Sit on an exercise bench, forearms resting on top of your thighs, wrists just beyond your knees; hold a barbell, using a pronated (thumbs in) grip (A).

Concentric phase: Lift the bar as high as possible, moving only at the wrist joint (B).

Eccentric phase: Slowly lower the bar to the starting position.

Variations: 1. Place forearms across an exercise bench.
2. Use dumbbells.

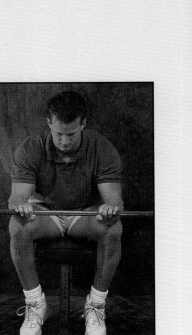

Back

Barbell

Dumbbell

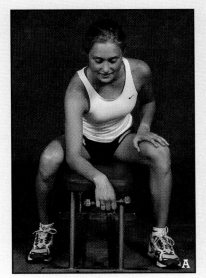

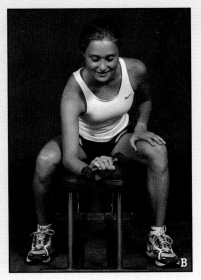

Leg Exercises

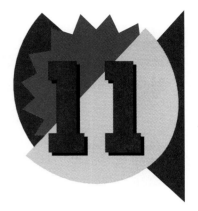

◀ Hip and Knee Extension (Gluteus maximus, Quadriceps, Hamstrings)
- ◀ Barbell Squat
- ◀ Dumbbell Squat or Dead Lift
- ◀ Barbell Squat in Power Rack
- ◀ Dead Lift

- ◀ Universal Squat Machine
- ◀ Cybex Leg Press Machine
- ◀ Nautilus Leg Press Machine
- ◀ Universal Leg Press Machine

- ◀ Lunge
- ◀ Step Up
- ◀ Leg Press Machine
- ◀ Hack Squat Machine

◀ Hip Extension (Gluteus maximus)
- ◀ Cybex Hip Extension Machine

◀ Hip Flexion (Illiopsoas)
- ◀ Cybex Hip Flexion Machine

◀ Knee Extension (Quadriceps)
- ◀ Universal Leg Extension Machine
- ◀ Body Master Leg Extension Machine

◀ Knee Flexion (Hamstrings)
- ◀ Nautilus Seated Leg Curl
- ◀ Body Master Leg Curl

◀ Ankle Plantar Flexion
- ◀ Standing Barbell Calf Raise
- ◀ Standing Dumbbell Calf Raise
- ◀ Universal Heel Raise
- ◀ Cybex Standing Calf Raise Machine

- ◀ One-Dumbbell Calf Raise
- ◀ Calf Press on Body Master Leg Press Machine
- ◀ Calf Press on Cybex Leg Press Machine
- ◀ Seated Calf Raise

HIP AND KNEE EXTENSION

SQUAT

Muscles developed: Quadriceps, gluteus maximus, hamstrings, erector spinae.

Starting position: Stand holding a barbell across your shoulders and upper back (A).

Eccentric phase: Inhale as you bend your knees and hips while keeping your head up and your back flat. Continue bending your knees and hips until your thighs are parallel to the floor (B).

Concentric phase: Exhale as you straighten your legs and hips to return to a standing position.

Spotting: Have one spotter stand directly behind you, or have one spotter at each end of the bar. If no spotters are available, use a squat rack to guarantee that you will not get stuck under a heavy weight.

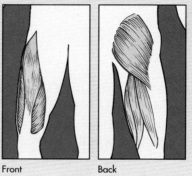

Front   Back

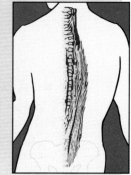

Back

Barbell

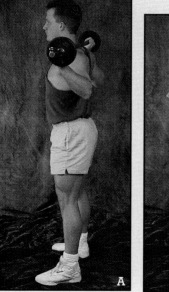

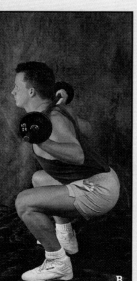

Dumbbell Squat or Deadlift

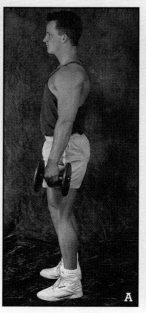

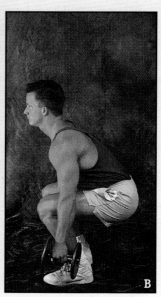

BARBELL SQUAT IN POWER RACK

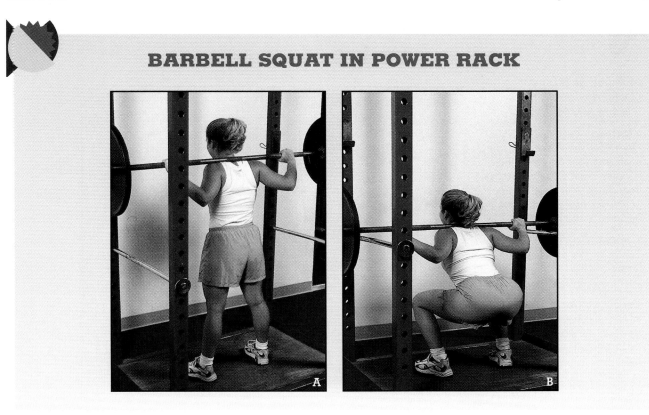

DEAD LIFT

Muscles developed: Erector spinae, gluteus maximus, quadriceps, hamstrings, trapezius, rhomboids, finger flexors.

Starting position: Bend over and assume a mixed grip on a barbell that is lying on the floor. Bend your knees and hips so your hips are approximately knee level or parallel to the floor. Hold your head up and your back straight (A).

Concentric phase: Keep your neck and back straight while you pull up on the bar (B). Lift the weight by extending your hips and knees.

Eccentric phase: Keep your neck and back straight as you slowly lower the weight back to the floor by bending your knees and hips.

Additional information: The dead lift is basically a hand-held squat. Because your leg muscles are much larger and stronger than your back extensor muscles and other upper body muscles, it is extremely important to maintain correct exercise position and progress slowly to avoid injury. Performed correctly, this is an excellent exercise to strengthen your back extensor muscles as well as your hip and knee extensors.

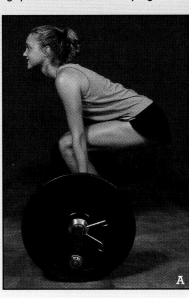

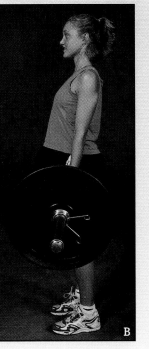

UNIVERSAL SQUAT

Muscles developed:
Quadriceps, gluteus maximus, hamstrings, erector spinae.

Starting position:
Place your shoulders under the pads and your hands on the handles located on the exercise bars. Keep your head up and your back straight with your hips and knees bent (A).

Concentric phase:
Exhale as you extend your knees and hips while keeping your back straight (B).

Eccentric phase:
Inhale as you lower the weight slowly to the starting position by bending your knees and hips.

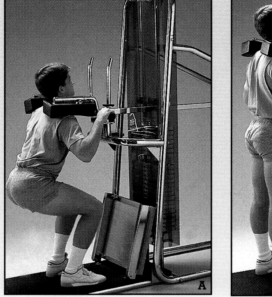
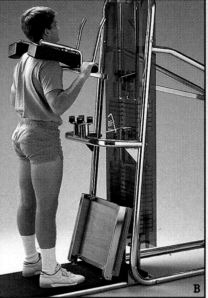

CYBEX LEG PRESS

Muscles developed: Quadriceps, gluteus maximus.

Starting position: Start on your back with your shoulders against the pads, your feet on the platform shoulder-width apart, and your knees bent at a 90° angle (A).

Concentric phase: Exhale as you extend your knees and hips (B).

Eccentric phase: Inhale as you bend your knees and hips and slowly return to the starting position.

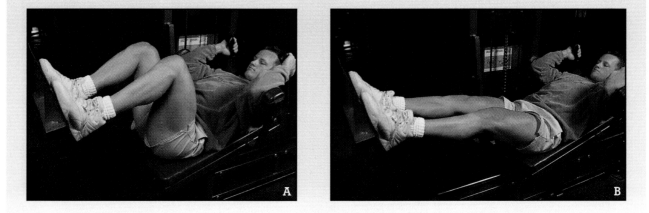

NAUTILUS LEG PRESS

Muscles developed: Quadriceps, gluteus maximus.

Starting position: Start in a sitting position with your knees bent at a 90° angle (A).

Concentric phase: Exhale as you extend your legs (B).

Eccentric phase: Inhale as you bend your legs slowly and allow the weight to return to the starting position.

Additional information: This exercise provides back support and therefore takes the strain off the spinal column but it will not strengthen the back extensor muscles like the barbell squat and dead lift.

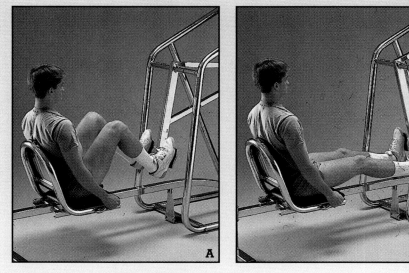

UNIVERSAL LEG PRESS

Muscles developed:
Quadriceps, gluteus maximus.

Starting position:
Start in a sitting position
with your knees bent at a
90° angle (A).

Concentric phase:
Exhale as you extend your
legs (B).

Eccentric phase:
Inhale as you slowly bend your
legs and allow the weight to
return to the starting position.

Additional information:
This exercise provides back
support and therefore takes the
strain off of the spinal column
but will not strengthen the back extensor muscles like the barbell squat and dead lift.

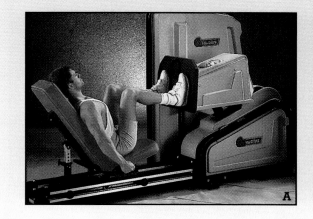

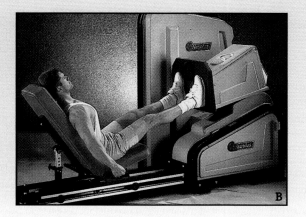

LUNGE

Muscles developed:
Quadriceps, gluteus maximus.

Starting position:
Assume a standing position with a dumbbell in each hand (A), or a barbell across your shoulders and upper back.

Eccentric phase:
Inhale as you take a large step forward with one leg. Bend the knee of your forward leg, and lower your body until the thigh of the front leg is parallel to the floor (B). (This is essentially a one-leg parallel squat.)

Concentric phase:
Exhale as you extend your forward leg, pushing yourself back to your original standing position.

Spotting:
Spotting is not necessary if you are doing lunges with dumbbells. If you are doing lunges with a barbell across your back and shoulders, have one spotter stand at each end of the bar. Or perform the lunges into a squat rack that could support the weight in case you cannot return to the standing position.

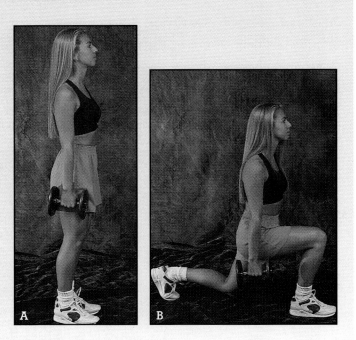

Additional information: Keep your head up and upper body erect throughout the exercise.

STEP UP

Muscles developed:
Quadriceps, gluteus maximus.

Starting position:
Take a standing position with a dumbbell in each hand (A), or a barbell across your upper back and shoulders.

Concentric phase:
Place one foot on the step in front of you. Using your hip and leg muscles, lift yourself up until your leg is straight (B).

Eccentric phase:
Lower yourself slowly to the starting position using the same leg.

Spotting:
If using dumbbells, you should be all right without a spotter. When using a barbell, have one spotter stand behind you, or a spotter at each end of the bar.

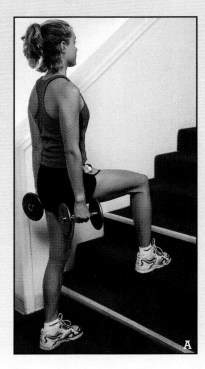
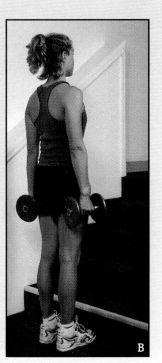

LEG PRESS

HACK SQUAT

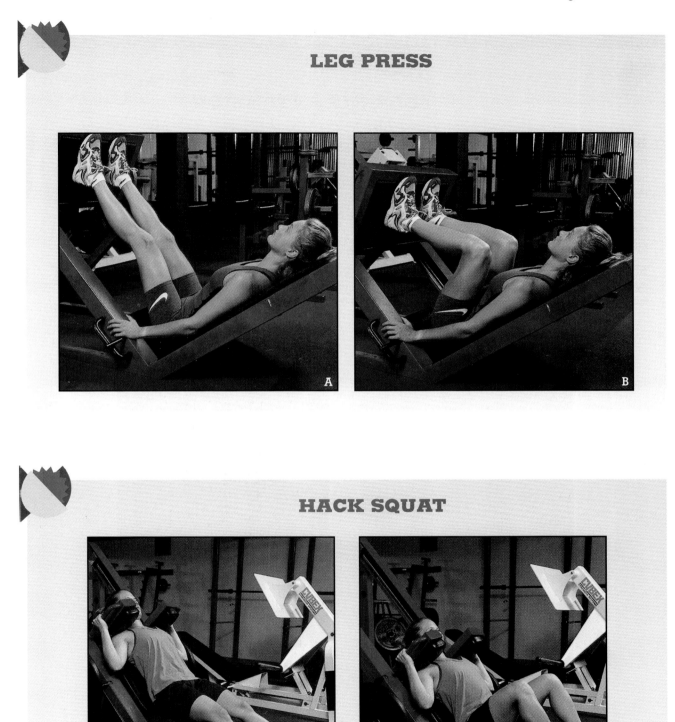

HIP EXTENSION

CYBEX HIP EXTENSION

Muscles developed: Gluteus maximus, hamstrings.

Starting position: Start in a standing position with one leg over the padded exercise bar, your hands holding the stability bar, and your hip joint lined up with the point of rotation of the exercise machine (A).

Concentric phase: Exhale as you pull your thigh down and back (hip extension) against the resistance (B).

Eccentric phase: Inhale as you slowly allow your leg to return to the starting position.

Additional information: If you keep your knee bent throughout the exercise, your gluteus maximus muscle will do most of the lifting. If you straighten your knee as you extend your hip, the hamstrings will be in a better position to help with hip extension.

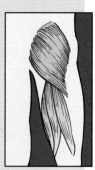

Back

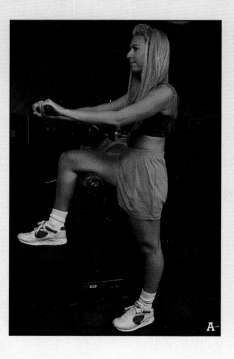

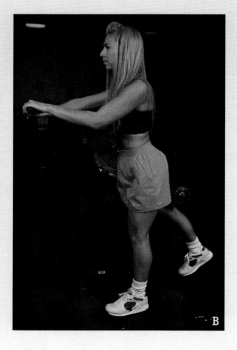

HIP FLEXION

CYBEX HIP FLEXION

Muscles developed: Iliopsoas, rectus femoris.

Starting position: Start in a standing position with one leg against the padded exercise bar and both hands holding the stability bar. The padded exercise bar should be just above your knee joint. Your hip joint should be lined up with the point of rotation of the exercise machine (A).

Concentric phase: Exhale as you pull your bent leg upward against the resistance (B). Tighten your abdominal muscles and keep your lower back flat.

Eccentric phase: Inhale as you lower your leg slowly to the starting position.

Caution: The hip flexors exert a strong pull forward on the lower portion of the spinal column. Therefore, it is important to stabilize the lower spinal column by flexing the abdominal muscles. This exercise is not recommended for individuals with weak abdominal muscles.

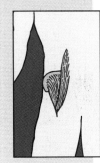

Back

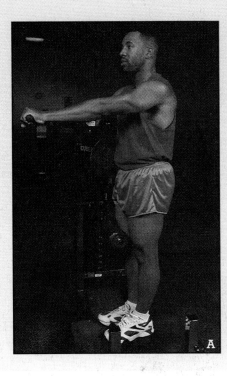

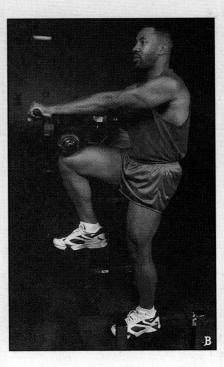

KNEE EXTENSION

Muscles developed: Quadriceps.

Starting position: Start in a seated position with your knees bent and the padded exercise bar in front of your ankle or lower leg. Grasp the handles located on each side of the machine (A).

Concentric phase: Exhale as you extend your legs at the knee joints (B). Pause at the extended position but do not go beyond extension.

Eccentric phase: Inhale as you slowly allow your legs to bend and return to the starting position.

Caution: Control the exercise movement. Do not hyperextend your knee joint. Do not allow the weight to drop.

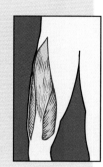

Front

UNIVERSAL LEG EXTENSION MACHINE

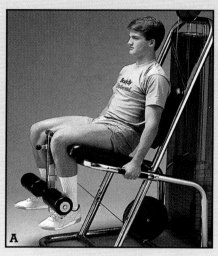

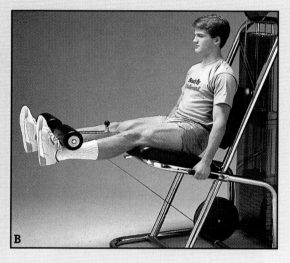

BODY MASTER LEG EXTENSION

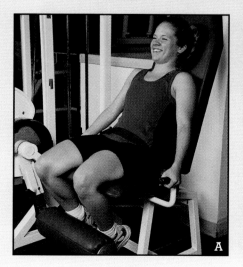

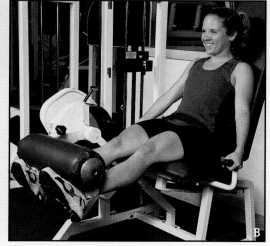

KNEE FLEXION

Muscles developed: Hamstrings.

Starting position: Start in a sitting or lying position with your legs straight and the back of your lower leg against the padded exercise bar. Line up your knees with the pivot point of the exercise machine. Grasp the handles. On the seated leg curl, fasten the seat belt to hold your hips in the correct exercise position (A).

Concentric phase: Exhale as you bend your knees and pull your lower legs toward the back of your thighs (B).

Eccentric phase: Inhale as you allow your legs to slowly return to the starting position.

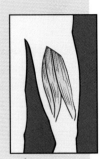

Back

NAUTILUS SEATED LEG CURL

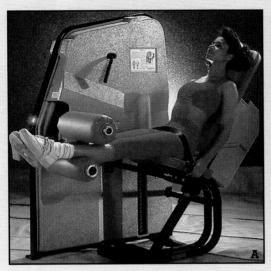

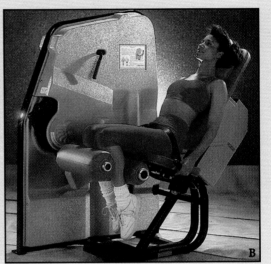

BODY MASTER LEG CURL

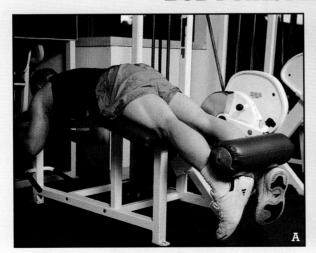

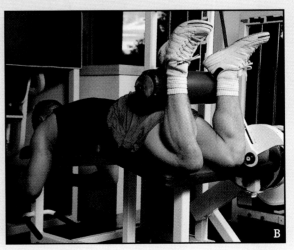

ANKLE PLANTAR FLEXION

STANDING CALF RAISE

Muscles developed: Gastrocnemius, soleus.

Starting position: Take a standing position with a barbell across your shoulders and upper back, the front half of both feet elevated so that your heels are lower than your toes (A).

Concentric phase: Exhale while moving only at the ankle joint to raise your heels as high as possible (B). Pause briefly, and completely contract the muscles on the back of your legs when you are at the highest position you can reach.

Eccentric phase: Inhale as you slowly lower both heels as far as they can go. The best stretch and maximum range of motion are achieved if your heels cannot touch the floor at the bottom position of this exercise.

Additional information: Maintaining balance is difficult during this exercise. Performing the exercise in a power rack or on a standing calf-raise machine usually increases the effectiveness of the exercise because it eliminates the balance problem.

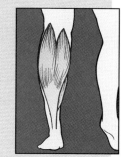

Back

Barbell

Dumbbell

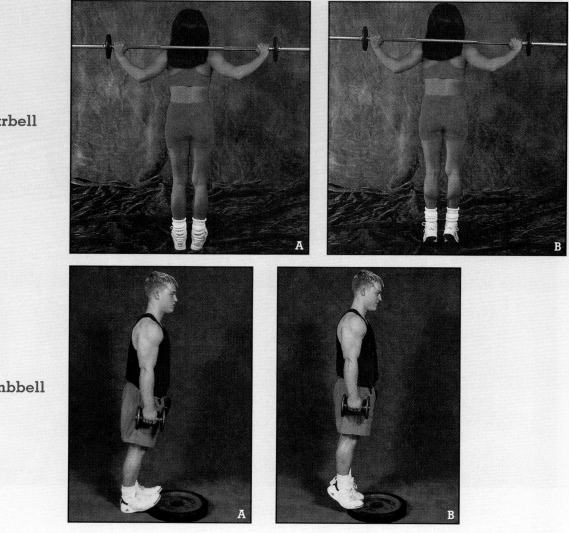

UNIVERSAL HEEL RAISE

CYBEX STANDING CALF RAISE MACHINE

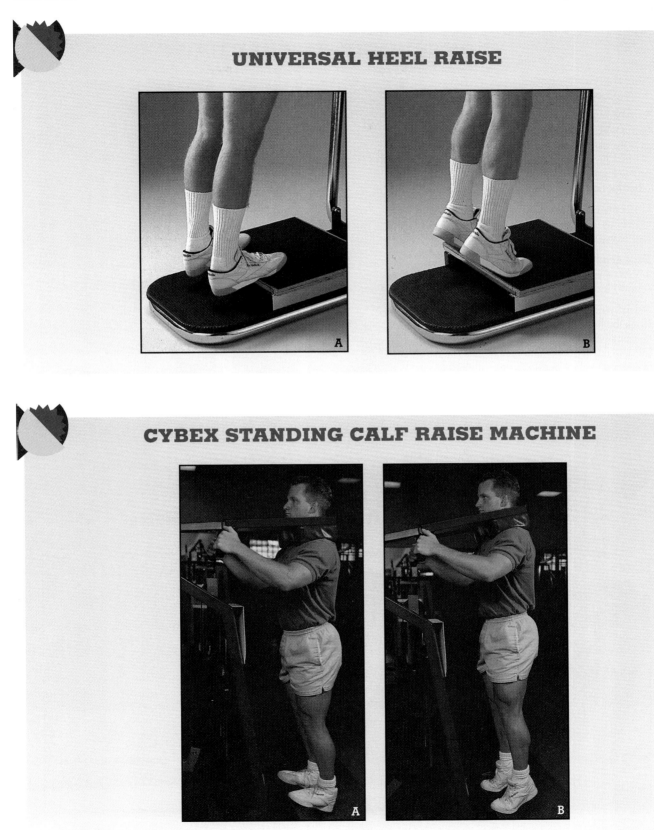

ONE-DUMBBELL CALF RAISE

Muscles developed:
Gastrocnemius, soleus.

Starting position:
Stand with a dumbbell in one hand hanging at arms length and resting against the side of your thigh. Place all of your body weight on the leg nearest the dumbbell and lift your other foot off the floor (A).

Concentric phase:
Exhale as you raise the heel of your support foot as high as possible. Pause at the top.

Eccentric phase:
Inhale as you slowly lower the heel of your support foot to a fully stretched position.

Additional information:
Place the hand that is not holding the dumbbell on some solid support for balance (B). Use the support hand for balance only; do not pull with that arm to help lift the weight.

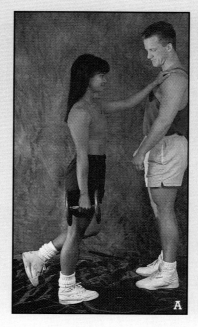

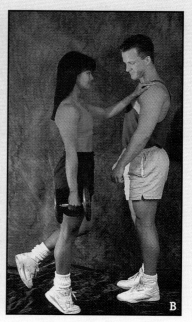

CALF PRESS
ON BODY MASTER LEG PRESS MACHINE

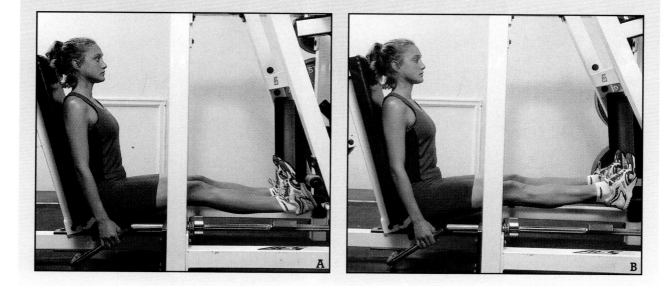

CALF PRESS ON CYBEX LEG PRESS

Muscles developed: Gastrocnemius, soleus.

Starting position: Position yourself on a leg press machine. Start with your legs straight, the front half of each foot on the pedals or platform, and your heels lower than the front part of your foot (A).

Concentric phase: Exhale as you press down with the front part of your foot moving only at the ankle joint (B). At the top of your range of motion, hold the muscle contraction and squeeze with your calf muscles.

Eccentric phase: Inhale as you slowly return to the starting position. Stretch the calf muscles in the starting position by allowing the heels to sink as low as possible.

Caution: Do **not** allow your feet to slip off the pedals or platform.

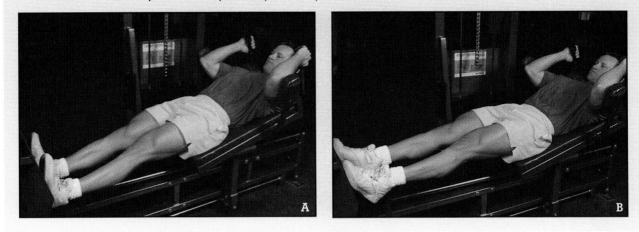

SEATED CALF RAISE

Muscles developed:
Soleus (the gastrocnemius becomes much less effective at pulling up on your heel when your knee is bent).

Starting position:
Sit with the front half of your foot on the foot plate, your knees under the padded exercise bar, and your hands on top of the exercise bar. Your heels should be lower than the front part of your foot (A).

Concentric phase:
Lift your heels as high as possible while keeping the front part of your foot on the foot plate (B).

Eccentric phase:
Slowly lower your heels to the starting position and stretch.

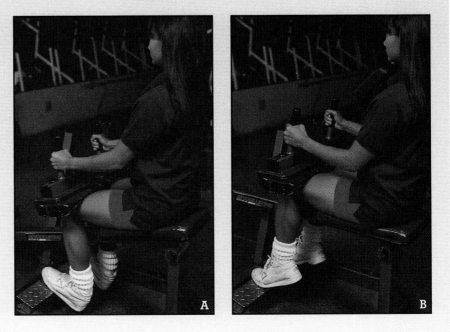

Abdominal and Back Extension Exercises

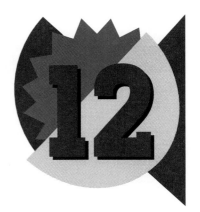

■ **Trunk Flexion (Abdominals)**
- Crunches, Curl-Ups
- Cybex Abdominal Machine
- Nautilus Abdominal Crunch Machine

■ **Trunk and Hip Flexion (Abdominals and Hip flexors)**
- Sit-Ups
- Tuck Ups
- Reverse Crunches
- Seated Reverse Crunches
- Hanging Reverse Crunches or Hanging Knee Raises

■ **Trunk Extension (Erector spinae)**
- Back Extension
- Universal Seated Back Extension Machine
- Cybex Back Extension Machine

TRUNK FLEXION (Abdominals)

CRUNCHES, CURL-UPS

Muscles developed: Rectus abdominis, abdominal obliques.

Starting position: Start flat on your back. Bend at your knees and hips. Place your feet flat on the floor. Cross your arms over your chest, with each hand touching the opposite shoulder (A).

Concentric phase: Exhale as you "curl up" slowly, pulling your head, neck, shoulders, and upper back off the floor in that order (B). Keep your lower back on the floor throughout the exercise. At the upper limit of this movement, "crunch" or squeeze the abdominal muscles by holding this fully contracted position for 3 seconds.

Eccentric phase: Slowly release the curling motion, and inhale as you return to the starting position.

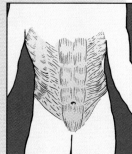

Front

Variations:

1. Keeping your legs straight, place the back of your legs against a wall, with your hips flexed and your back on the floor.

2. Place your lower legs up on a bench with your hips and knees bent.

3. Add a twisting motion to the trunk flexion so that as you curl up, you also move one elbow toward the opposite hip. Alternate the direction of the twist on each repetition.

Additional information: If you want to add weight to this exercise, place it on your upper chest and hold it there by crossing your arms on top of the weight. Or hold a weight in your hands directly above your shoulders with your arms straight. Push the weight straight up toward the ceiling as you curl your trunk.

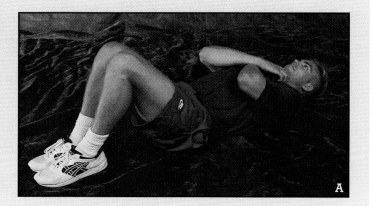

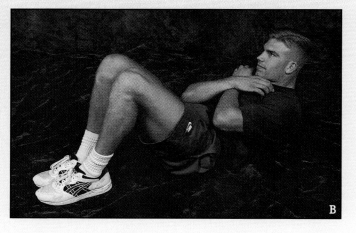

CYBEX ABDOMINAL MACHINE

Muscles developed:
Rectus abdominis, abdominal obliques.

Starting position:
Start in a seated position with your feet under the anchor straps and your upper chest against the padded exercise bar (A).

Concentric phase:
Exhale as you pull with your abdominal muscles to curl your chest toward your hips (B).

Eccentric phase:
Inhale as you slowly allow your chest to return to the starting position.

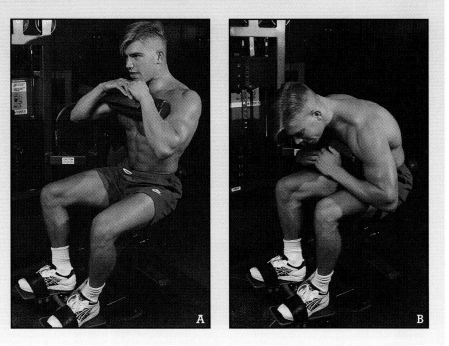

NAUTILUS ABDOMINAL CRUNCH MACHINE

Muscles developed: Rectus abdominis, abdominal obliques.

Starting position: Start in a seated position with your upper back against the padded exercise bar. Fasten the seat belt and grasp the handles on the exercise bar.

Concentric phase: Exhale as you pull with your abdominal muscles to curl your chest toward your hips.

Eccentric phase: Inhale as you slowly allow your chest to return to the starting position.

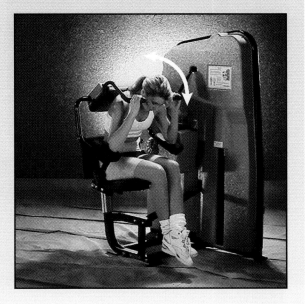

TRUNK AND HIP FLEXION (Abdominals and Hip Flexors)

SIT-UPS

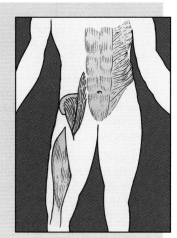

Front

Muscles developed: Rectus abdominis, iliopsoas, abdominal obliques, rectus femoris.

Starting position: Start flat on your back with your knees bent and both feet flat on the floor; place your fingertips on the opposite shoulder (A).

Concentric phase: Exhale as you slowly pull your head, neck, shoulders, upper back, and lower back off the floor, in that order (B).

Eccentric phase: Slowly return to the starting position by placing your lower back, upper back, shoulders, neck, and head back on the floor, in that order. Inhale as you near the starting position.

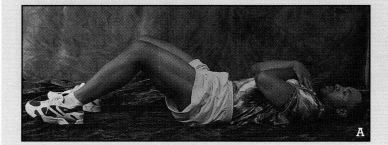

Variations:

1. Twisting sit-ups (require trunk flexion and trunk rotation). Curl up and twist, touching one elbow to the opposite knee. Alternate the direction of the twist on each repetition.
2. Change your arm position, or add weight. If you add weight, place it on your upper chest and hold it in place with your hands.

As weight is added, you probably will have to anchor your feet by placing them under something or by having someone hold them.

Additional information: This exercise requires the use of the hip flexors near the end of the concentric phase of the exercise, which does not seem to be a problem if the trunk is fully flexed first.

Caution: Do **not** pull with the hip flexor muscles until the abdominal muscles are fully contracted. Do not pull on your head with your arms.

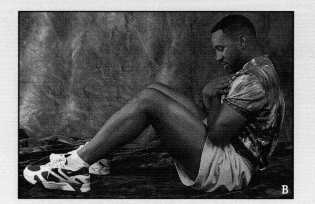

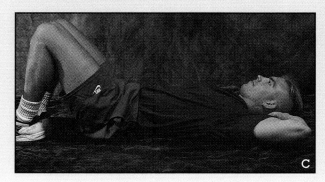

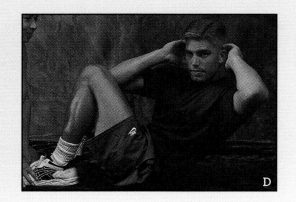

TUCK-UPS

Muscles developed:
Rectus abdominis, abdominal obliques, iliopsoas.

Starting position:
Start on your back with your legs extended and your arms extended overhead (A).

Concentric phase:
Exhale as you flex your trunk, hips, and knees while bringing your arms and chest toward your legs. Finish in a tucked sitting position (B).

Eccentric phase:
Inhale as you return slowly to the starting position.

Variations:
The "V Sit-Up": Keep your arms and legs extended as you raise them, and touch your fingers to your toes as they reach the top of the upward motion.

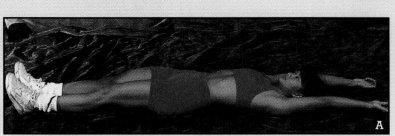
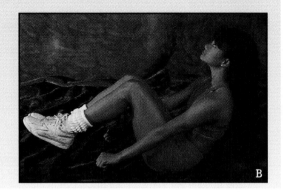

REVERSE CRUNCHES

Muscles developed: Rectus abdominis, abdominal obliques.

Starting position: Start on your back, and bend your hips and knees so that your feet are flat on the floor; place your arms by your sides (A).

Concentric phase: Exhale as you slowly pull your knees toward your shoulders. Lift your hips and lower back off the floor. Focusing on the abdominal muscles, pull the pelvic girdle toward the rib cage (B).

Caution: Do not roll back on your head and neck; stay on your upper back and shoulders.

Eccentric phase: Inhale as you slowly return to the starting position.

Variations:

1. Start with your legs straight. Pull your heels toward your hips first, then pull your knees toward your shoulders.

2. Twisting reverse crunches. Try to pull one knee toward the opposite shoulder. Alternate the direction of the twist on each repetition.

Caution: Perform this exercise in a controlled manner. Vigorous twisting of the trunk can result in injury to the spinal column.

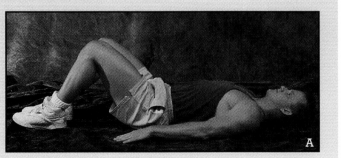
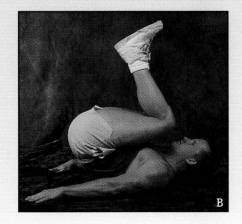

SEATED REVERSE CRUNCHES

Muscles developed: Rectus abdominis, abdominal obliques, iliopsoas.

Starting position: Sit on the edge of a bench or chair. Lean back with your shoulders, straighten your legs, and lift both feet off of the floor (A).

Concentric phase: Exhale as you bring your knees up toward your shoulders (B).

Eccentric phase: Inhale as you return your legs slowly to the starting position.

Variations:

1. Keep your hips and knees bent throughout the exercise. From this position with your legs tucked up, curl or crunch the pelvic girdle toward the rib cage, then return to the starting position but do not extend at the knee or hip joints.

2. Follow variation 1, except twist the torso so that you pull one shoulder toward the opposite knee. Alternate the twisting motion on each repetition.

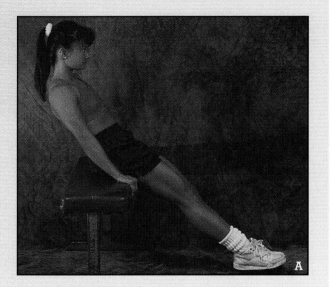

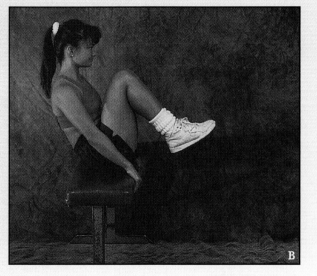

HANGING REVERSE CRUNCH OR KNEE RAISES

Muscles developed: Rectus abdominis, abdominal obliques, iliopsoas.

Starting position: Hang from your hands (A).

Concentric phase: Exhale as you bring your knees up toward your shoulders (B).

Eccentric phase: Inhale as you return your legs slowly to the starting position.

Variations:

1. Lift your knees up and keep them up while you do abdominal crunches.
2. Add a twisting motion near the completion of the knee raise so that one knee is pulled toward the opposite shoulder. Alternate the twisting motion on each repetition.

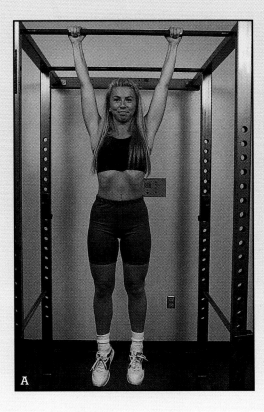

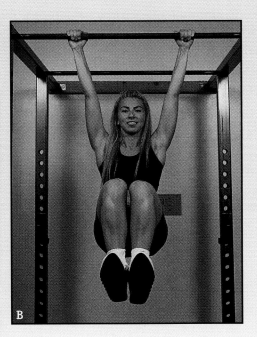

TRUNK EXTENSION (Erector spinae)

BACK EXTENSION

Muscles developed: Erector spinae.

Starting position: Start on a flat exercise bench with the front of your legs and hips on the bench and with your upper body beyond the end of the bench (A). Have someone hold your feet.

Concentric phase: Inhale as you raise your upper body to a position in which your back is parallel to the floor (B).

Eccentric phase: Exhale as you return slowly to the starting position.

Additional information: You may use a specially designed back extension bench if you have one available.

Variations:

1. Place your hands on your lower back.

2. Cross your arms on your chest

3. Place your hands behind your head. As your arms move away from your waist and toward your head, the resistance increases.

4. If you wish to add additional resistance, hold a barbell plate behind your neck or on your chest.

Caution: Perform this exercise in a smooth and controlled manner. Raising your head and shoulders above parallel and arching your back is not recommended.

Back

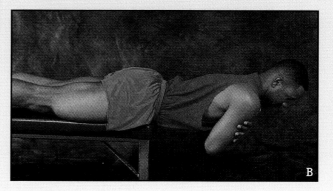

A

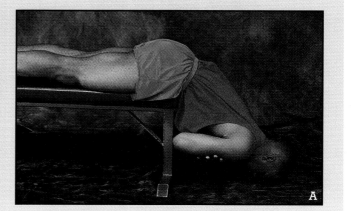

B

UNIVERSAL SEATED BACK EXTENSION MACHINE

Muscles developed:
Erector spinae.

Starting position:
Start in a seated position leaning forward with your feet under the padded stability bar and your hands holding onto the handles on the side of the seat (A). Your upper back should be against the padded exercise bar.

Concentric phase:
Inhale as you press backward and extend your back (B).

Eccentric phase:
Exhale as you return slowly to the starting position.

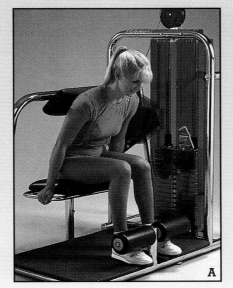
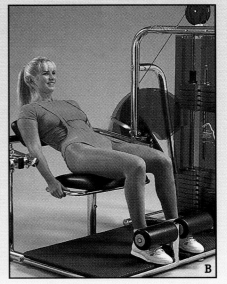

CYBEX BACK EXTENSION MACHINE

Muscles developed:
Erector spinae.

Starting position:
Start in a seated position, leaning forward with your feet on the foot plate. Cross your arms on your chest or place your hands on the front of your thighs (A). Your upper back should be against the padded exercise bar.

Concentric phase:
Inhale as you press backward and extend your back (B).

Eccentric phase:
Exhale as you return slowly to the starting position.

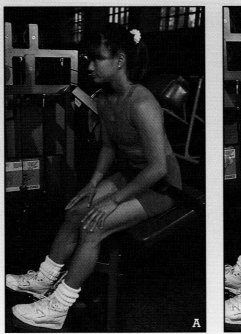
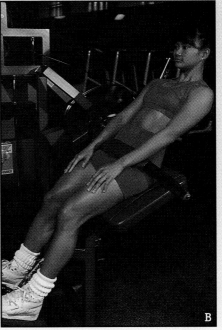

THE AB SOLUTION

"How can I get rid of this?" is a common question that is asked frequently while pointing to a protruding abdomen. If you want to reduce your waist circumference there are three things you need to work on. You probably already know the first two, but the last one might surprise you.

1. Reduce your stored body fat level.
2. Increase your abdominal muscle strength and muscle tone.
3. Improve your posture.

If you have excess body fat on your abdomen, you probably already know what you need to do. Burn more calories than you consume. Eat healthy, but eat less than you do now. Increase your aerobic activity to burn more calories per day. And finally, engage in a progressive resistance exercise program (weight training) to build more muscle, which will increase your metabolic rate.

Your abdomen might also be bulging because of weak abdominal muscles. See the earlier part of this chapter for exercises to strengthen your abdominal muscles and follow the exercise guidelines in this book.

You have probably heard all of the above ideas many times. You also know it takes a long time to see any change. If you would like to reduce your waist by two inches immediately, try this. Stand up straight, lift your chest, pull your shoulders back, and pull your abdomen in.

Poor posture is a major contributing factor for a protruding abdomen. To reinforce good posture, add the following exercises to your regular weight-training program.

1. Perform deep-breathing straight-arm pull-overs with a light to moderate weight to lift and stretch your rib cage. Refer to the chapter on chest exercises to learn how to perform this exercise.

2. Perform a rowing exercise with a moderate weight with an emphasis on squeezing your elbows together and pulling your shoulders back in the fully contracted position. Hold this position for one to three seconds on each repetition to develop the muscles that pull your shoulders back. Refer to the chapter on back exercises to learn how to perform rowing exercises.

3. Perform a back extension exercise to develop the erector spinae muscles, which, as the name implies, erect the spine and pull the spine into good posture. Refer to the back extension exercises in this chapter.

4. For a few minutes each day, probably in a private place, put a hardbound book on the top of your head and practice standing, sitting, and walking with good posture.

The **AB SOLUTION** is a combination of reducing your stored body fat, increasing your abdominal muscle strength, and improving your posture.

Nutrition, Rest, and Drugs

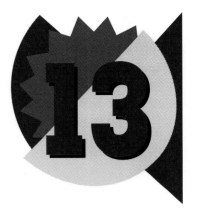

NUTRITION

The average American will spend approximately 6 years of his or her life eating. That will include about 70,000 meals and 60 tons of food. Sound dietary practices will help you maintain a high level of health throughout your life.

The nutrients your body needs to function properly can be divided into six categories.

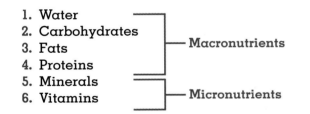

1. Water
2. Carbohydrates
3. Fats — Macronutrients
4. Proteins
5. Minerals
6. Vitamins — Micronutrients

The nutrients in these six categories provide most of the chemicals necessary for your body to:

- produce energy,
- grow and develop new tissue,
- repair damaged tissue,
- conduct nerve impulses,
- reproduce, and
- regulate physiological processes.

Water

Water contains no calories or vitamins, yet it is essential in relatively large quantities for your body to function properly. Approximately 60%–70% of your body weight is water, yet most people seldom think about the importance of adequate water intake. You might live up to 50 days without food, but without water you would likely die from dehydration in less than a week.

When you are thirsty, your body is asking for water (H_2O). However, thirst is not always an accurate indicator of your need for water. You should drink at least 8 to 10 glasses of water a day. Factors such as your size, activity level, environment, and diet affect your need for water intake.

What do you give your body when you are thirsty? Not all fluids contribute to your water needs. In fact, some beverages (coffee, tea, and alcohol) actually dehydrate your body and increase your need for additional water.

It would be difficult for you to drink too much water. If you do happen to take in more than your body needs, you can get rid of any excess easily. You lose water every day in urine, feces, sweat, and through evaporation from your lungs.

If you do not take in enough water, your body cannot continue to function normally. Your health and performance will suffer.

Minerals

Minerals are inorganic substances that are necessary for some of the chemical activity that goes on in your body. If the appropriate minerals are not present, certain chemical changes cannot occur. Minerals are essential in regulating body functions such as muscle contraction, protein synthesis, and heart function. Approximately 25 minerals are considered essential for sustaining life.

The major minerals that your body needs include calcium, phosphorus, magnesium, sodium, potassium, and chloride. Because they are found in a variety of foods, mineral deficiencies are not common in people who are eating a balanced diet. The one exception is calcium. A National Academy of Sciences study found that 80% of the women over age 18 who were surveyed consumed too little calcium. A calcium deficiency can cause osteoporosis (a thinning of the bones).

Trace minerals, those you need in small amounts, include iron, zinc, copper, fluoride, and selenium. Even though trace minerals are required only in small amounts, they are still essential for your health. Some women do not get enough iron. A survey by the U.S. Department of Agriculture discovered that many women between ages 19 and 50 get only about 60% of the iron they need each day. This can lead to iron-deficiency anemia. Eating a balanced diet is the safest way to prevent mineral deficiencies. Table 13.1 shows the major functions of minerals in the body.

Vitamins

Vitamins are organic substances that are necessary for some of the chemical activity that goes on in your body. Vitamins do not contain calories and therefore do not directly supply energy. However, they are necessary to release the energy stored in carbohydrates, fats, and proteins. They are also necessary for tissue building and controlling your body's use of food.

You need 13 vitamins. The two major categories of vitamins are: fat-soluble (A, D, E, K) and water-soluble (C and the eight B-complex vitamins). Since fat-soluble vitamins can be stored in your body, you can take in too much of these. Excess water-soluble vitamins are normally excreted in the urine. A toxic effect can occur when certain vitamins are taken in excessive amounts. Therefore, it's generally healthier to get your vitamins from a balanced diet instead of vitamin supplements.

Table 13.2 lists the vitamins, their functions, and foods that contain them.

Your body needs adequate amounts of water, minerals, and vitamins. A deficiency will decrease optimal bodily function and performance. However,

TABLE 13.1 Major Functions of Minerals

Nutrient	Good Sources	Major Functions	Deficiency Symptoms
Calcium	Milk, yogurt, cheese, green leafy vegetables, dried beans, sardines, and salmon	Required for strong teeth and bone formation. Maintenance of good muscle tone, heartbeat, and nerve function	Bone pain and fractures, periodontal disease, muscle cramps
Iron	Organ meats, lean meats, seafoods, eggs, dried peas and beans, nuts, whole and enriched grains, and green leafy vegetables	Major component of hemoglobin. Aids in energy utilization	Nutritional anemia, and overall weakness
Phosphorus	Meats, fish, milk, eggs, dried beans and peas, whole grains, and processed foods	Required for bone and teeth formation. Energy release regulation	Bone pain and fracture, weight loss, and weakness
Zinc	Milk, meat, seafood, whole grains, nuts, eggs, and dried beans	Essential component of hormones, insulin, and enzymes. Used in normal growth and development	Loss of appetite, slow healing wounds, and skin problems
Magnesium	Green leafy vegetables, whole grains, nuts, soybeans, seafood, and legumes	Needed for bone growth and maintenance. Carbohydrate and protein utilization. Nerve function. Temperature regulation	Irregular heartbeat, weakness, muscle spasms, and sleeplessness
Sodium	Table salt, processed foods, and meat	Body fluid regulation. Transmission of nerve impulse. Heart action	Rarely seen
Potassium	Legumes, whole grains, bananas, orange juice, dried fruits, and potatoes	Heart action. Bone formation and maintenance. Regulation of energy release. Acid-base regulation	Irregular heartbeat, nausea, weakness
Selenium	Seafood, meat, whole grains	Component of enzyme; functions in close association with vitamin E	Muscle pain, possible heart muscle deterioration; possible hair and nail loss

TABLE 13.2 Major Functions of Vitamins

Nutrient	Good Sources	Major Functions	Deficiency Symptoms
Vitamin A	Milk, cheese, eggs, liver, and yellow/dark green fruits and vegetables	Required for healthy bones, teeth, skin, gums, and hair. Maintenance of inner mucous membranes, thus increasing resistance to infection. Adequate vision in dim light.	Night blindness, decreased growth, decreased resistance to infection, rough-dry skin
Vitamin D	Fortified milk, cod liver oil, salmon, tuna, egg yolk	Necessary for bones and teeth. Needed for calcium and phosphorus absorption	Rickets (bone softening), fractures, and muscle spasms
Vitamin E	Vegetable oils, yellow and green leafy vegetables, margarine, wheat germ, whole grain breads and cereals	Related to oxidation and normal muscle and red blood cell chemistry	Leg cramps, red blood cell breakdown
Vitamin K	Green leafy vegetables, cauliflower, cabbage, eggs, peas, and potatoes	Essential for normal blood clotting	Hemorrhaging
Vitamin B_1 (Thiamine)	Whole grain or enriched bread, lean meats and poultry, organ fish, liver, pork, poultry, organ meats, legumes, nuts, and dried yeast	Assists in proper use of carbohydrates. Normal functioning of nervous system. Maintenance of good appetite.	Loss of appetite, nausea, confusion, cardiac abnormalities, muscle spasms
Vitamin B_2 (Riboflavin)	Eggs, milk, leafy green vegetables, whole grains, lean meats, dried beans and peas	Contributes to energy release from carbohydrates, fats, and proteins. Needed for normal growth and development, good vision, and healthy skin	Cracking of the corners of the mouth, inflammation of theskin, impaired vision.
Vitamin B_6 (Pyridoxine)	Vegetables, meats, whole grain cereals, soybeans, peanuts, and potatoes	Necessary for metabolism of protein and fatty acids and normal red blood cell formation	Depression, irritability, muscle spasms, nausea
Vitamin B_{12}	Meat, poultry, fish, liver, organ meats, eggs, shellfish, milk, and cheese	Required for normal growth, red blood cell formation, nervous system and digestive tract functioning	Impaired balance, weakness, drop in red blood cell count
Niacin	Liver and organ meats, meat, fish, poultry, whole grains, enriched breads, nuts, green leafy vegetables, and dried beans and peas	Contributes to energy release from carbohydrates, fats, and proteins. Normal growth and development, and formation of hormones and nerve-regulating substances	Confusion, depression, weakness, weight loss
Biotin	Liver, kidney, eggs, yeast, legumes, milk, nuts, dark green vegetables	Essential for carbohydrate metabolism and fatty acid synthesis	Inflamed skin, muscle pain, depression, weight loss
Folic Acid	Leafy green vegetables, organ meats, whole grains and cereals, and dried beans	Needed for cell growth and reproduction and red blood cell formation	Decreased resistance to infection
Pantothenic Acid	All natural foods, especially liver, kidney, eggs, nuts, yeast, milk, dried peas and beans, and green leafy vegetables	Related to carbohydrate and fat metabolism	Depression, low blood sugar, leg cramps, nausea, headaches
Vitamin C (Ascorbic Acid)	Fruits and vegetables	Helps protect against infection; formation of collagenous tissue. Normal blood vessels, teeth, and bones	Slow healing wounds, loose teeth, hemorrhaging, rough-scaly skin, irritability

the results of independent research to date have indicated that more than the required amount does not improve performance or progress. A good guideline to follow is to eat a balanced diet from a variety of good foods and to drink at least 8 to 10 glasses of water a day.

Carbohydrates

Calories (body fuel) are contained in carbohydrates, fats, and proteins. (See Figure 13.1.) Carbohydrates are a major source of energy for your body, particularly during high-intensity exercise. Each gram of carbohydrate contains approximately 4 calories.

Simple carbohydrates, sometimes referred to as simple sugars, tend to have little nutritive value. Foods such as cookies, soft drinks, and candy are high in simple sugars and are often eaten instead of more nutritious foods.

Complex carbohydrates provide your body with many of the valuable nutrients needed to keep you healthy. These complex carbohydrates are found primarily in foods from plant sources such as breads, fruits, vegetables, rice, pasta, and cereals. The exception is milk, which is the only significant animal source.

Fats

Fats (lipids) are the most concentrated source of energy at 9 calories per gram. That is more than twice

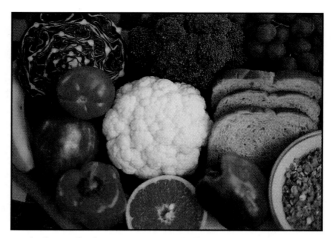

A balanced diet is essential for maintaining good health.

the calories in a gram of carbohydrates or proteins. Fats have a higher energy value than carbohydrates and provide up to 70% of your energy needs when you are in a resting state or during low-level physical activity. Fats are also an essential component of cell walls and nerve fibers. They are involved in absorbing and transporting fat-soluble vitamins, supporting and cushioning organs, and insulating your body.

Although fats are useful in your body, it is possible to have too much of a good thing. Excess fat in your diet contributes to high blood pressure, heart disease, diabetes, and other diseases. Too much body fat is a risk factor for heart disease and has been associated with certain cancers (colon, breast, prostate, and uterus).

Since the correct amount of fat is good and too much is bad, what you need is the right amount of fat in your diet. The American Heart Association and the U. S. Department of Health and Human Services recommend that less than 30% of your daily calories come from fats. Fats should not be cut completely out of your diet, nor should you eat too many fats. Either extreme can be detrimental.

There are different categories of fats, but saturated fats require special mention because of their associated risk of cardiovascular disease. Saturated fats contribute to an increase in blood cholesterol levels. Your cholesterol level is affected more by the percent of fat in your diet than by the cholesterol you eat. Elevated blood cholesterol is a major risk factor for heart disease. Less than 10% of your

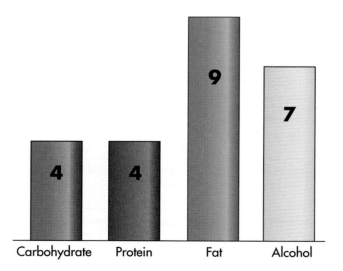

Carbohydrate   Protein   Fat   Alcohol

Source: *Principles and Labs For Fitness & Wellness* by Werner W. K. Hoeger and Sharon A. Hoeger. Morton Publishing Company, 1997, pg. 39.

FIGURE 13.1 Caloric value of food.

total daily caloric intake should come from saturated fats. Figure 13.2 shows the fat content of selected foods.

Proteins

Proteins are complex organic compounds made up of amino acids. They are essential for growth and

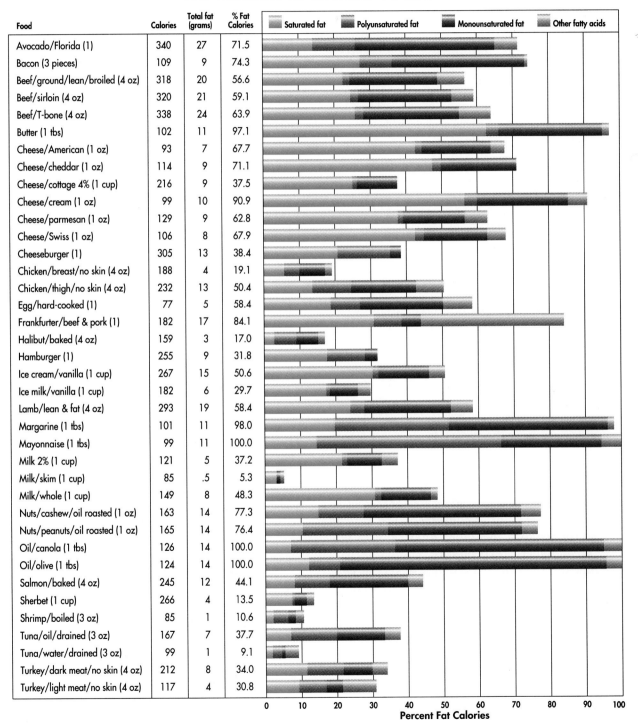

FAT CONTENT OF SELECTED FOODS

Food	Calories	Total fat (grams)	% Fat Calories
Avocado/Florida (1)	340	27	71.5
Bacon (3 pieces)	109	9	74.3
Beef/ground/lean/broiled (4 oz)	318	20	56.6
Beef/sirloin (4 oz)	320	21	59.1
Beef/T-bone (4 oz)	338	24	63.9
Butter (1 tbs)	102	11	97.1
Cheese/American (1 oz)	93	7	67.7
Cheese/cheddar (1 oz)	114	9	71.1
Cheese/cottage 4% (1 cup)	216	9	37.5
Cheese/cream (1 oz)	99	10	90.9
Cheese/parmesan (1 oz)	129	9	62.8
Cheese/Swiss (1 oz)	106	8	67.9
Cheeseburger (1)	305	13	38.4
Chicken/breast/no skin (4 oz)	188	4	19.1
Chicken/thigh/no skin (4 oz)	232	13	50.4
Egg/hard-cooked (1)	77	5	58.4
Frankfurter/beef & pork (1)	182	17	84.1
Halibut/baked (4 oz)	159	3	17.0
Hamburger (1)	255	9	31.8
Ice cream/vanilla (1 cup)	267	15	50.6
Ice milk/vanilla (1 cup)	182	6	29.7
Lamb/lean & fat (4 oz)	293	19	58.4
Margarine (1 tbs)	101	11	98.0
Mayonnaise (1 tbs)	99	11	100.0
Milk 2% (1 cup)	121	5	37.2
Milk/skim (1 cup)	85	.5	5.3
Milk/whole (1 cup)	149	8	48.3
Nuts/cashew/oil roasted (1 oz)	163	14	77.3
Nuts/peanuts/oil roasted (1 oz)	165	14	76.4
Oil/canola (1 tbs)	126	14	100.0
Oil/olive (1 tbs)	124	14	100.0
Salmon/baked (4 oz)	245	12	44.1
Sherbet (1 cup)	266	4	13.5
Shrimp/boiled (3 oz)	85	1	10.6
Tuna/oil/drained (3 oz)	167	7	37.7
Tuna/water/drained (3 oz)	99	1	9.1
Turkey/dark meat/no skin (4 oz)	212	8	34.0
Turkey/light meat/no skin (4 oz)	117	4	30.8

Legend: Saturated fat · Polyunsaturated fat · Monounsaturated fat · Other fatty acids

Percent Fat Calories

FIGURE 13.2 Saturated fat, monounsaturated fat, and polyunsaturated fat content of selected foods.

repair of body tissues. Proteins are a potential source of energy but are not normally used for fuel when carbohydrates and fats are available.

Of the 20 amino acids that have been identified, nine are essential in your diet. A food that contains all nine essential amino acids is called a complete protein food. Foods from animal sources such as meat, eggs, and milk provide complete proteins. Incomplete proteins come from plant sources such as beans, peas, and nuts.

If any one of the amino acids is missing, your body cannot put together all of the protein structures it needs, including muscle tissue.

Carbohydrates, fats, and proteins are all necessary in your daily food intake. In each case, a deficiency creates a problem, an adequate amount is optimal, and more is not better. The suggested caloric intake balance for adults as shown in Figure 13.3 is:

55% to 60% from carbohydrates,
Less than 30% from fats, and
10% to 20% from proteins.

THE "SECRET" WEIGHT TRAINING DIET

Many weight trainers and athletes are looking for the "secret" or "magic" diet that will make them successful and produce miraculous results. The truth is, no one food or special diet will do that. The "secret" diet is a balanced diet that includes all of the nutrients your body needs in the correct amounts.

The only major difference between the diet that is best for the average sedentary adult and the diet that is best for the active athlete or weight trainer is the total number of calories consumed. The athlete or weight trainer may use more total calories because of greater energy expenditure.

The fundamental principles of the "secret" weight training diet are moderation, variety, and balance. Your diet should include a wide variety of good quality food in the proper amounts. You must eat right to gain healthy muscle tissue and remove excess stored body fat. Choose foods that are high in nutrients compared to their calories. These are referred to as foods with "high nutrient density." Foods that have few nutrients and are high in calories are referred to as "junk foods." Carbonated drinks and chips will not produce quality muscle tissue but certainly can be

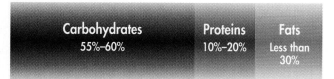

FIGURE 13.3 A balanced diet.

stored as fat. Remove the junk food from your diet and eat high quality foods. Learn to tell the difference. One of the top body builders in the world has claimed that his body building success was 80% nutrition and 20% training.

One relatively easy way to balance all of your complex nutritional requirements is to follow the U. S. Department of Agriculture's Food Guide Pyramid (Figure 13.4). The pyramid translates nutrient recommendations into a food group plan. This plan guides you to a balanced intake of essential nutrients. It is based on a recommended number of servings from six food groups.

1. 6 to 11 servings daily from the bread, cereal, rice, and pasta group.

2. 3 to 5 servings daily from the vegetable group.

3. 2 to 4 servings daily from the fruit group.

4. 2 to 3 servings daily from the milk, yogurt, and cheese group.

5. 2 to 3 servings daily from the meat, poultry, fish, dry beans, eggs, and nuts group.

6. Sparingly (use very little) from the fats, oils, and sweets group.

The Food Guide Pyramid is a general guide, not an exact prescription, to healthy eating. However, knowing the recommendations from the pyramid should help you in making healthy food choices for a diet that is right for you. Also refer to Figure 13.4 to assist in making healthy food choices.

The following are eating guidelines from the United States Department of Agriculture:

1. Maintain a healthy body weight.

2. Eat a variety of foods.

3. Emphasize grains, fruits, and vegetables in your diet.

4. Eat a low-fat, low-cholesterol diet.

5. Eat sugars sparingly.

6. Limit salt intake.

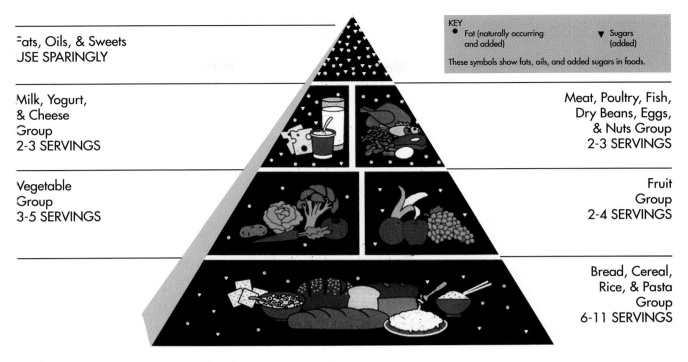

Fats, Oils, & Sweets
USE SPARINGLY

KEY
● Fat (naturally occurring and added)   ▼ Sugars (added)
These symbols show fats, oils, and added sugars in foods.

Milk, Yogurt,
& Cheese
Group
2-3 SERVINGS

Meat, Poultry, Fish,
Dry Beans, Eggs,
& Nuts Group
2-3 SERVINGS

Vegetable
Group
3-5 SERVINGS

Fruit
Group
2-4 SERVINGS

Bread, Cereal,
Rice, & Pasta
Group
6-11 SERVINGS

What counts as one serving?

Breads, Cereals, Rice, and Pasta
1 slice of bread
1/2 cup of cooked rice or pasta
1/2 cup of cooked cereal
1 ounce of ready-to-eat cereal

Vegetables
1/2 cup of chopped raw or cooked vegetables
1 cup of leafy raw vegetables

Fruits
1 piece of fruit or melon wedge
3/4 cup of juice
1/2 cup of canned fruit
1/4 cup of dried fruit

Milk, Yogurt, and Cheese
1 cup of milk or yogurt
1½ to 2 ounces of cheese

Meat, Poultry, Fish, Dry Beans, Eggs, and Nuts
2½ to 3 ounces of cooked lean meat, poultry, or fish
Count 1/2 cup of cooked beans, or 1 egg, or 2 tablespoons of peanut butter as 1 ounce of lean meat (about 1/3 serving)

Fats, Oils, and Sweets
LIMIT CALORIES FROM THESE
especially if you need to lose weight

The amount you eat may be more than one serving. For example, a dinner portion of spaghetti would count as two or three servings of pasta.

A Closer Look at Fat and Added Sugars

The small tip of the Pyramid shows fats, oils, and sweets. These are foods such as salad dressings, cream, butter, margarine, sugars, soft drinks, candies, and sweet desserts. Alcoholic beverages
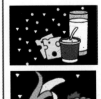
are also part of this group. These foods provide calories but few vitamins and minerals. Most people should go easy on foods from this group.

Some fat or sugar symbols are shown in the other food groups. That's to remind you that some foods in these groups can also be high in fat and added sugars, such as cheese or ice cream from the milk group, or french fries from the vegetable group. When choosing foods for a healthful diet, consider the fat and added sugars in your choices from all the food groups, not just fats, oils, and sweets from the Pyramid tip.

How many servings do you need each day?

	Women & some older adults	Children, teen girls, active women, most men	Teen boys & active men
Calorie level*	about 1,600	about 2,200	about 2,800
Bread group	6	9	11
Vegetable group	3	4	5
Fruit group	2	3	4
Milk group	2–3**	2–3**	**2–3
Meat group	2, for a total of 5 ounces	2, for a total of 6 ounces	3, for a total of 7 ounces

* These are the calorie levels if you choose lowfat, lean foods from the 5 major food groups and use foods from the fats, oils, and sweets group sparingly.

** Women who are pregnant or breastfeeding, teenagers, and young adults to age 24 need 3 servings.

*Developed by the U.S. Department of Agriculture to promote a healthy diet for people in the United States.

FIGURE 13.4 The Food Guide Pyramid.

7. Drink alcoholic beverages in moderation or not at all.

Use the food logs at the end of this chapter to keep track of what you eat for 3 days. Compare your diet to the recommendations on the Food Guide Pyramid.

NUTRIENT SUPPLEMENTATION

If you are eating according to the recommendations of the United States Department of Agriculture (USDA) Food Guide Pyramid you will be consuming a balanced diet of high quality foods that should meet all of your nutritional needs. Independent researchers (those who do not sell food supplements) have found no benefit from the use of supplements when subjects were on a healthy diet that was meeting all of their nutritional needs.

If you have dietary deficiencies, supplements might be beneficial. However, it would be healthier to improve your diet first before resorting to "quick fix" supplements to make up for your poor eating habits. *Weight training for life* encourages a lifelong pattern of healthy, balanced exercise supported by healthy balanced eating.

WEIGHT GAIN

To gain muscular body weight, perform brief heavy weight training workouts. Work the largest muscles in your body and eat a balanced diet of high quality foods. Increase your total caloric intake by 500 to 1,000 calories per day. Eat smaller meals and

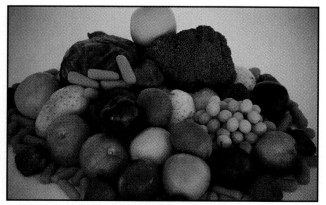

A balanced diet should include plenty of fruits and vegetables.

more frequently. Get plenty of rest. Slow down, stay calm, and decrease your other activities. Set a healthy goal to gain muscle and not just total body weight. Watch your body fat level. Any diet in which caloric intake exceeds caloric need can lead to fat storage and unhealthy weight gain.

WEIGHT LOSS

Concerns about losing weight are increasing for many Americans. These concerns may be justified. According to the National Center for Health Statistics, 58 million people — one out of every three men and women — are obese and weigh at least 20% more than they should. The average weight for adults between the ages of 25 and 30 rose an amazing 10 pounds in just seven years — from 161 pounds in 1986 to 171 pounds in 1993.

At any given time, 33 to 40 percent of women and 20 to 24 percent of men are trying to lose weight. Another 28 percent of all adults are trying to maintain a weight loss — usually without success. The simple and well-documented truth is that diets are not an effective weight loss strategy. Only about 10% of the people who begin a diet without exercise are able to lose the desired weight. Only one in 200 is able to maintain the weight loss for any significant amount of time. Diets don't work.

So what is the key to weight management? The formula is to maintain a moderate level of total calories, minimize fat calories, and get a lot of exercise. A well-rounded exercise program including aerobic exercise, weight training, and flexibility activities is best for weight management and overall fitness.

Continuous, rhythmic activities that use large muscle groups are best for high-caloric expenditure. Examples of good fat-loss activities are walking, cycling, and jogging.

How does weight training fit into a fat loss program? When you start a weight training program, you will gain muscle and lose fat. Any significant loss in total body weight is difficult to attain until muscle growth slows down. To lose excess body fat, you should perform longer training sessions consisting of more sets, repetitions, and exercises, which will use more total calories. You cannot "spot reduce" body fat. For example, sit-ups do not "spot reduce" fat from the abdominal area.

Weight training increases lean body mass. Because of the high energy needs of muscle tissue, more calories are required just to maintain muscle tissue. Lean body mass has such an important role in metabolism that the maintenance of muscle tissue causes increased caloric expenditure even when you are not exercising. Weight training increases lean body mass (muscle), which in turn increases metabolic rate. This results in a greater caloric expenditure. Because weight training increases muscle mass (calorie burning cells), it is also beneficial for people who are at their recommended body weight but have a higher than recommended percentage of body fat.

An added benefit of weight training is the firm and fit appearance that results from regular training. Muscle tissue is more dense than fat tissue. Increasing muscle tissue and decreasing fat tissue results in a trim, healthy, toned appearance.

The secret to healthy weight loss is found in the following:

1. Eat a balanced diet of good quality food.
2. Do not skip meals or omit any particular food group.
3. Decrease your total caloric intake by 500 to 1000 calories per day.
4. Increase your physical activity level.
5. Select activities where food is not easily available.
6. Decrease the amount of rest and sleep you get. Your metabolic rate and caloric expenditure are lower when you are resting and sleeping.

REST

Weight training exercise is the stimulus, but the positive changes that occur in the muscular system as a result of weight training take place between exercise sessions as your body rebuilds and adapts to the exercise overload. Adequate rest and nutrition are necessary for these positive changes to occur.

Weight training progress is best when a muscle receives 2 to 4 days of rest between exercise sessions. Fewer than 2 days of rest or more than 4 days of rest between exercise sessions results in slower progress.

An average amount of sleep is 8 hours per night. However, sleep requirements vary from one person to another, and for the same person based upon changes in activity levels. Beginning weight trainers initially may find they need to sleep more to recover from this new demand. As they become

accustomed to the increased physical activity and their bodies begin to function more efficiently, they often return to normal sleep patterns.

"Hard gainers" — individuals who have a hard time gaining muscle — sometimes need as many as 10 hours of sleep each night. Some "easy gainers" or natural mesomorphs may gain on 7 hours of sleep per night. Not getting adequate rest is often one of the greatest obstacles to weight training progress for young adults. Many high school students, college students, and young adults train hard with weights but do not get enough sleep to recover completely from their training sessions.

Weight training is intense and demanding. Too many other physical activities will slow your weight training progress. If you want to maximize your weight training gains, you should cut down on other physically strenuous activities. Young adults (ages 16 to 30) are usually the ones who wear themselves out with a large number of activities. This combination of too much activity and not enough rest can cancel out all the hard work you put into your weight training exercises.

Some experienced weight trainers believe that they progress better if they train hard for 6 to 8 weeks, take one week off, then start a new training program.

As you get older, some of your bodily functions will naturally begin to slow down. You should not view this as a totally negative experience. Many older adults report that they need less sleep, less food, and less exercise to stay healthy and physically fit. Beyond an approximate age of 40 or 50, two weight training workouts per week might be sufficient to maintain the muscular system in excellent condition. This depends on your weight training goals and your personal ability to recover from your workouts.

Some days you feel better than others. There undoubtedly will be days when you will not feel like doing your normal workout. On those days you probably should train anyway but reduce your intensity and your total workload. You should not skip workouts completely on those days. Frequency of workouts should be maintained. Once you skip a training session, it becomes easier to skip another and another until soon you have no training schedule at all. It is easy to stop training completely and difficult to get started again. Many will begin weight training, but few will have what it takes to continue for the rest of their lives. Persistence is a common word but a rare human quality.

The only time you should not train is when you are sick or injured. If you are truly physically sick, you should not work out, because it will further stress your body. You cannot "sweat out" a cold or any other illness. Instead, you should follow your doctor's advice and rest completely so you can get well in the shortest possible time. If you keep training, an illness can drag on for weeks, and you probably will not experience any progress in spite of your training efforts. Weight training should contribute to your health. When you are not well, you should stop training and get well, then start again. If you are sick more than two or three times a year, you should examine your lifestyle.

If you feel exhausted when you wake up and are sleepy all day long, even during activities you normally enjoy, you may not be getting enough rest. If you are sleeping about 8 hours each night but are still feeling tired, you may be overtraining. In that case, you might try reducing the total number of sets in your weight training program and see if you feel better.

Adequate rest and recovery time are essential to your weight training progress.

DRUGS

Anabolic Steroids

Anabolic steroids present the biggest drug problem in weight training. They are synthetic compounds that are like the natural hormones your body produces. Most of the steroids that weight trainers and athletes use to gain muscle mass are similar to the hormone testosterone.

These anabolic steroids are thought to promote muscle growth, but they have been difficult to study because they also produce highly undesirable and dangerous side effects. Therefore, they can be studied only at safe (low) levels. The athletes who claim that steroids work take massive doses, at least 10 to 20 times greater than the safe dose an ethical physician would allow in a research study with human subjects.

Steroid use is dangerous because serious, life-threatening side effects and adverse reactions can occur (see Figure 13.5). The side effects for female

steroid users are just as dangerous as they are for men. Some of the undesirable side effects that have been reported by users and observed by doctors include: endocrine disturbances, atrophy of the testicles, male impotency, liver damage, liver cancer, psychological disturbances, and coronary artery disease.

All steroid users agree that steroids work only when accompanied by extremely hard weight training. Therefore, steroids are not an "easy gain" muscle drug that replaces hard work. Intense workouts are still necessary to gain muscle. This is another reason steroid effects are hard to study. It is difficult to determine how much of the improvement is a result of training and how much can be attributed to the steroid effect.

Many steroid users have reported an increase in aggressiveness. This can result in more intense weight training workouts, which might produce greater gains by itself.

Because anabolic steroids do not produce scientifically proven and predictable benefits, and they do have documented and dangerous side effects, their use is not recommended. Some young lifters and body builders who are taking steroids are causing lifelong damage to their bodies that they will regret when they get older. Steroid abuse also has caused a number of deaths.

Weight training is an activity that should improve your health and natural performance level. Drug abuse has no place in a health development program such as *weight training for life*.

Alcohol

Although there is no evidence that a low level of alcohol consumption interferes with weight training progress, there is also no evidence that it has any beneficial effect on your weight training progress. Heavy alcohol consumption does have profound detrimental effects on your body (Figure 13.6). If your desire is to have a strong and healthy body, you need to keep your alcohol consumption to a minimum or eliminate it completely.

Tobacco

Smoking or chewing tobacco has no known beneficial effects. Smoking is harmful to the respiratory and circulatory systems (Figure 13.7). It decreases your performance and training capacity. Smoking will reduce your ability to complete demanding weight training workouts and will interfere with your ability to recover from your workouts. Smoking and chewing tobacco both have been proven to cause cancer and other diseases, and neither will help you reach your weight training goals.

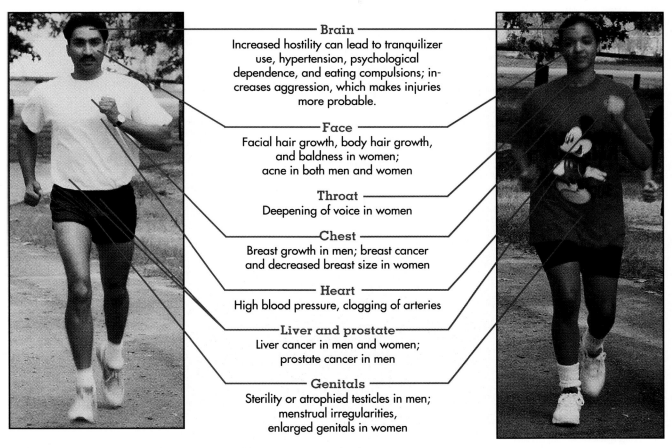

Brain
Increased hostility can lead to tranquilizer use, hypertension, psychological dependence, and eating compulsions; increases aggression, which makes injuries more probable.

Face
Facial hair growth, body hair growth, and baldness in women; acne in both men and women

Throat
Deepening of voice in women

Chest
Breast growth in men; breast cancer and decreased breast size in women

Heart
High blood pressure, clogging of arteries

Liver and prostate
Liver cancer in men and women; prostate cancer in men

Genitals
Sterility or atrophied testicles in men; menstrual irregularities, enlarged genitals in women

FIGURE 13.5 Adverse effects of steroids on parts of the body.

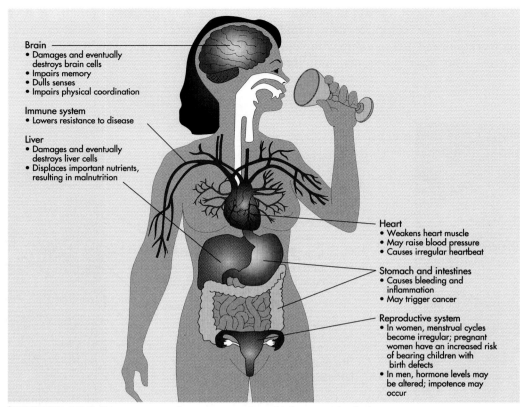

FIGURE 13.6 Long-term risks associated with chronic alcohol use.

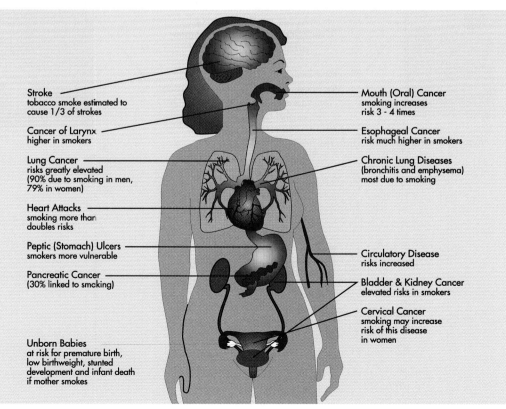

FIGURE 13.7 Adverse health effects of smoking.

FOOD DIARY

Name _____ Date _____ Total Caloric Intake: _____

Time	Place	Associated Activity	Reason/Mood	Food and Amount	Dairy	Meat	Grain	Vegs	Fruits	Fats	Misc.	Water
Breakfast												
Snack												
Lunch												
Snack												
Dinner												
Snack												
Exercise												

Food Groups

FOOD DIARY

Name _____ Date _____ Total Caloric Intake: _____

Time	Place	Associated Activity	Reason/Mood	Food and Amount	Dairy	Meat	Grain	Vegs	Fruits	Fats	Misc.	Water
Breakfast												
Snack												
Lunch												
Snack												
Dinner												
Snack												
Exercise												

FOOD DIARY

Name　　　　　　　　　　　　　　Date　　　　　　Total Caloric Intake:

Time	Place	Associated Activity	Reason/Mood	Food and Amount	Food Groups							
					Dairy	Meat	Grain	Vegs	Fruits	Fats	Misc.	Water
Breakfast												
Snack												
Lunch												
Snack												
Dinner												
Snack												
Exercise												

FOOD DIARY

Name _____ Date _____ Total Caloric Intake: _____

	Time	Place	Associated Activity	Reason/Mood	Food and Amount	Dairy	Meat	Grain	Vegs	Fruits	Fats	Misc.	Water
Breakfast													
Snack													
Lunch													
Snack													
Dinner													
Snack													
Exercise													

Food Groups

Record-Keeping and Progress

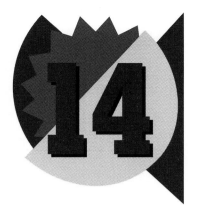

RECORD KEEPING

It is important to keep track of your progress by recording each training session. Write down what you do during each workout as soon as you have done it.

Weight training is not an exact science. Although some general guidelines have evolved for weight training, many variables affect your progress, and these can be changed. Every individual is different and therefore responds differently to a weight training stimulus. The information you record during your training sessions can be a valuable source of information about your personal response to a variety of weight training programs. You will be able to look back through your records and compare your progress with your training methods. This should help you find which exercises and training methods work best for you.

The important things to record are:

☑ The name of each exercise.

☑ The order in which exercises are performed.

☑ The resistance used in each set.

☑ The repetitions completed in each set.

☑ The day of the week.

☑ The date.

☑ Perhaps a general comment about how you felt or anything that might have influenced your training that day, positive or negative (for example, "felt tired, 2 hours sleep").

Keeping track of your weight training sessions helps to provide motivation and to ensure the correct exercise stimulus. From the written record of what you were able to do during the previous training session comes a challenge to do a little bit more — one more repetition or 5 more pounds. Figures 14.1 and 14.2 provide examples of written record keeping, the first informal and the second an easy-to-use form.

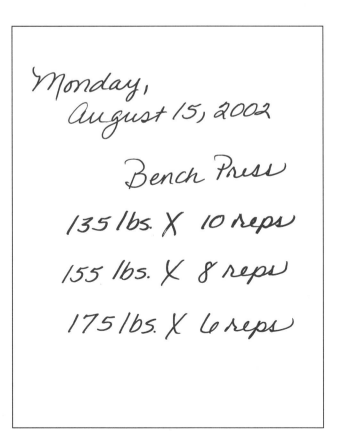

FIGURE 14.1 Open-page log.

STRENGTH AND MUSCULAR ENDURANCE PROGRESS LOG

Name: _____

Date	23 Sept 2005														
Exercise	Wt	Rep	Wt	Rep	Wt	Rep	Wt	Rep	Wt	Rep	Wt	Rep	Wt	Rep
Bench Press	135	10												
	155	8												
	175	6												

FIGURE 14.2 Sample form for record keeping.

MEASURING PROGRESS

Measuring Strength

Strength is the ability of a muscle to exert force. If you are training with weights to gain strength, you can measure your progress in at least two common ways: (1) workout repetition maximums, and (2) one repetition maximums. Weight training for maximum strength gain requires that you lift relatively heavy weight (85% to 100% of your one repetition maximum) for relatively low repetition maximums (1-RM to 6-RM). Your repetition maximum is the maximum amount of weight you can lift for a given number of repetitions. For example, if you can complete 5 repetitions with 155 pounds but cannot do another repetition, your 5-RM is 155 pounds. After a few more workouts, if you can complete 5 repetitions with 160 pounds, you have increased your strength as indicated by the increase in your 5-RM.

A second way to test your progress is by testing your one-repetition maximum (1-RM) periodically using the exercises you perform in your training program.

Your 1-RM is the heaviest weight you can lift one time while maintaining correct exercise technique. Of course, you will be limited to the heaviest weight you can lift through the weakest point in the range of motion. But you will still find the heaviest weight you can lift one time, and this is a measurement of your ability to exert force (strength).

The first time you test your 1-RM, start with a light weight and perform 10 repetitions to warm up. Then add weight to each subsequent set and perform one repetition in each set until you find the heaviest weight you can lift correctly one time. Try to find your 1-RM within five or six sets. To find your maximum strength, you need to perform enough sets for the muscles to be warmed up but not so many that the muscles are fatigued.

To perform 1-RM strength tests after the first time, start with a warm-up set of 10 repetitions with 60% of your previous 1-RM. Then perform one repetition each at 80%, 85%, 90%, and 95% of your previous 1-RM. After these progressively heavier sets, try for a new personal record based upon how the 95% load felt. If the 95% felt easy, you may want to try 10 pounds more than your previous 1-RM. If the 95% set was very hard,

you may want to try just 2½ pounds or 5 pounds more than your previous 1-RM. Rest about 2 minutes between each set, and 3 to 5 minutes before attempting your new personal record.

If you fail to maintain correct exercise form on a strength test so you can lift a heavier weight, you are lying to yourself about your true strength level.

You also have a greater risk of injury when you begin to perform exercises improperly to lift a greater weight than you can really handle.

Always use spotters for the exercises in which you could get trapped under a heavy weight. Do not try to perform 1-RMs in all of your exercises.

As a beginning weight trainer, you might want to test 1-RMs once a month for the first 6 to 12 months. After that, increases come more slowly, so testing once every 2 or 3 months might be adequate.

You also may choose never to test your 1-RM strength. If 1-RM strength is not important, interesting, or motivating to you, you probably have no reason to test it. There is no reason for you to risk injury or failure attempting 1-RM lifts if it is not important to you.

Measuring Muscular Endurance

Muscular endurance is the ability of a muscle to exert force for a long time or for many repetitions. If you are training with weights to gain muscular endurance, you can measure your progress by performing as many consecutive repetitions as possible with an established weight.

Select a weight that is at least 50% but not more than 70% of your 1-RM. Perform as many continuous repetitions as possible without any pause between repetitions. Maintain strict exercise form.

Repeat this test once a month using the same weight every time. An increase in the number of repetitions you can complete is evidence of an increase in your muscle endurance.

Measuring Size

The most common way to measure changes in muscle size is to measure the circumference of various body parts with a tape measure. Although circumference measurements include many other kinds of tissue (bone, fat, blood vessels, skin, and so on), muscle and fat are the two tissues that change the most. If you are training your muscles hard and eating properly, circumference gains should be a result of increased muscle and losses should be a result of decreased fat.

Have your training partner measure you or learn to measure yourself. A Gulick tape measure is ideal if one is available. A Gulick tape has a spring tension device on the end so that all measurements may be made with the same tension on the tape. If a Gulick tape is not available, measurements can be taken with a standard cloth tape measure. The tape should be placed around the circumference so that it is firm but not so tight that the skin is indented. Measure to the nearest eighth of an inch or half centimeter.

Measurements commonly taken by men and women who wish to change their appearance are listed here. These represent the circumference measurements that are most likely to change in response to a weight training program. For some body parts two measurements are described — relaxed and flexed. If you are trying to lose excess body fat, use the relaxed measurements. If you are trying to gain muscle size, use the flexed measurements. Take the measurements while you are in a standing position with your feet about 6" apart. The tape measure should be horizontal unless the directions for a body part specify something different.

Neck   *Relaxed*: Measure the horizontal circumference midway between the shoulders and the head.

Chest   *Relaxed*: Measure at the largest circumference during relaxed breathing. Do not lift your chest or flex your muscles.

Flexed (Expanded): Measure at the largest circumference of the chest with the lungs filled, rib cage lifted, and muscles flexed.

Waist   *Relaxed*: Measure the horizontal circumference at the level of the navel. The abdominal muscles should be in their normal state of tonus for a relaxed standing position.

Flexed: Measure the horizontal circumference with the abdomen pulled in as far as possible.

Hips   *Relaxed*: Measure at the largest horizontal circumference.

Flexed: Tighten the muscles in the hip region, and measure at the largest horizontal circumference.

For all of the following arm and leg measurements, hold the tape perpendicular to the limb segment being measured. Measure both arms and both legs.

Thigh   *Relaxed*: Measure the horizontal circumference midway between the hip joint and the knee joint.

Flexed: Slightly bend the knee joint, and contract all of the thigh muscles. Measure midway between the hip joint and the knee joint.

Calf or Leg   *Relaxed*: Measure at the largest circumference.

Flexed: Measure the largest circumference with the muscles of the leg flexed.

Upper Arm   *Relaxed*: With the arms hanging relaxed, measure the horizontal circumference midway between the shoulder joint and the elbow joint.

Flexed: Raise your arm to shoulder height and to the side of your body. Bend your elbow and flex all of the muscles of the upper arm. Measure the largest circumference.

Forearm   *Relaxed*: With your arm hanging in a normal relaxed position, measure the largest circumference of the forearm, between the wrist and the elbow.

Flexed: Bend your elbow and wrist so that as many forearm muscles as possible can be contracted. Measure at the largest circumference between the wrist and the elbow.

All of these measurements should be taken the first time you measure. After that you may choose to measure just the ones you are the most interested in. Beginning weight trainers might want to measure once a month for the first year. After the first year, changes tend to come more slowly, so you might want to take measurements once every 2 or 3 months.

The measurements suggested here are ones that are commonly used. Because they are used to measure your progress, muscle gain or fat loss, they should be taken exactly the same way each time and, if possible, with the same tape measure. These measurements are to provide information about the effectiveness of your training program.

Measuring Body Weight

If your goal is to change your body weight, this can be measured easily on an accurate scale. It is best to use the same scale, at the same time of day, wearing as little clothing as possible, and the same clothing each time. The scale measures total body weight but does not differentiate muscle and fat.

Measuring Body Fat

Skinfold measurements should be taken at the sites where you are most interested in losing excess body fat. There are standard measurement procedures for the different sites. These measurements should be taken by someone who is trained and experienced.

Photographs

Changes that take place in appearance are gradual and cannot be seen as they occur. Photographs of various poses can be an excellent means for periodically checking your progress. A photograph is the only way to really see yourself. Obviously the photograph should be taken while you are wearing as little clothing as possible, such as a swimsuit. Subsequent photographs should be taken with the same camera, location, position, and distance.

EVALUATING PROGRESS

Progress should not be checked too often. Physical changes take time. Beginners might be able to measure once a month and see progress, but more advanced weight trainers might check only once or twice a year.

Genetic Potential

Each individual has some upper limit on the amount of strength or size he or she can gain. For the beginning weight trainer, gains are relatively easy and fast. As progress continues and gains get close to a person's genetic limit, the gains become more difficult and slower.

One of the most intriguing aspects of weight training is that you have no way of knowing when you have reached your genetic limit, or if *anyone* has ever reached his or her limit. After years of weight training, body builders and strength athletes continue to improve, though the rate of improvement slows.

Problem Solving

When you have not made progress for a long time (2 or 3 months), problem solving is in order. What might be responsible for your lack of progress? Change the one thing that you think is the most likely cause of your lack of progress. Allow 3 or 4 weeks for the change to start making a difference. If no progress has occurred after a month, try changing a different variable. Give it time to work.

Changing more than one variable at a time may leave you with more questions than answers. Changing too often (less than 4 to 6 weeks) does not allow enough time to find out what works for you and what does not. Keep in mind that what works for you now may not work when your body adapts to it.

Some of the factors to consider in solving a lack of progress in weight training are:

- amount of resistance
- number of repetitions
- number of sets
- rest between sets
- number of exercises per body part
- total number of exercises performed
- order of exercises
- frequency of training
- concentration during exercise performance
- intensity of training
- regularity of training — hour and day

- motivation level
- nutrition
- rest
- other activities

- mental stress
- drugs
- alcohol
- tobacco

Name _____ Section_____

Size Measurement

Directions:

Read Chapter 14, Record Keeping and Progress, Size Measurement.

	1st Measurement Date:		2nd Measurement Date:		3rd Measurement Date:		4th Measurement Date:	
Height ⟶								
Weight ⟶								
Neck (relaxed) ⟶								
Chest (relaxed) ⟶								
(flexed) ⟶								
Waist (relaxed) ⟶								
(flexed) ⟶								
Hips (relaxed) ⟶								
(flexed) ⟶								
Right (R) Left (L)	R	L	R	L	R	L	R	L
Thigh (relaxed) ⟶								
(flexed) ⟶								
Calf (relaxed) ⟶								
(flexed) ⟶								
Upper Arm (relaxed) ⟶								
(flexed) ⟶								
Forearm (relaxed) ⟶								
(flexed) ⟶								

Name _____ Section _____

Strength Measurement

Directions:

1. Read the section "Measuring Strength," in Chapter 14, Record-Keeping and Progress.
2. Train with weights for at least 2 weeks before testing strength.
3. Test your strength every 4 weeks after the first test.
4. Move the weight in a smooth, continuous manner.
5. Maintain strict exercise form.
6. Do **not** hold your breath.
7. Increase the weight for each set.
8. Rest between sets.
9. Rest 3 to 5 minutes before your final record attempt.
10. Start with a light weight that you can lift 10 times. After that first warm-up set, continue increasing the weight and performing one repetition until you reach your one-repetition maximum (1-RM). Try to reach your 1-RM within five or six total sets.
11. Record the date, the exercise, and your 1-RM.
12. Always remember "Safety First." Don't injure yourself attempting 1-RM lifts.

Strength Test	1st Test	2nd Test	3rd Test	4th Test
	Date:	Date:	Date:	Date:
Exercise	Wt	Wt	Wt	Wt

Name _____ Section _____

Muscle Endurance Measurement

Directions:

1. Read the section "Measuring Muscular Endurance," in Chapter 14, Record Keeping and Progress.
2. Test your strength to find your one-repetition maximum.
3. Select a weight that is approximately 60% of your 1-RM.
4. Perform as many continuous repetitions as possible, with absolutely no rest pause between repetitions.
5. Move the weight in a smooth, controlled manner.
6. Maintain strict exercise form.
7. Test your muscle endurance every 4 weeks after the first test.
8. Use the same weight for each exercise every time you test yourself for muscle endurance on that exercise. An increase in repetitions using the same weight should indicate an increase in muscle endurance.

Muscle Endurance Test		1st Test Date:	2nd Test Date:	3rd Test Date:	4th Test Date:
Exercise	Weight	Reps	Reps	Reps	Reps

A Formula For Success

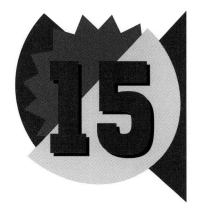

WHAT IS SUCCESS?

"Success" has a different meaning for each of us. In this chapter, success is defined as *setting a goal and achieving it*. Successful people achieve the goals they have set for themselves. A successful person reaches big success as a result of many smaller successes. Success breeds success. Achieving smaller goals that lead to larger ones is important. This process should result in a lifestyle that is as enjoyable as the attainment of each goal.

A FORMULA FOR SUCCESS

Written Goals

Goals are an extremely important part of any successful weight training program. Putting the necessary effort into weight training is difficult without some desirable goal to be reached. In addition to the motivation factor, a successful weight training program cannot be planned without a goal. All successful training programs are based on a desired outcome. If you don't have a desired outcome, how can you plan to reach it?

Goals should be as specific as possible. This may be difficult if you are just beginning a new activity such as weight training, but try to be as specific as possible.

Once you decide upon a goal, write it down. This is an important step. It is like making a contract with yourself. Your thoughts and spoken words tend to become modified with the passing of time, but your written goal will remain the same every time you read it. Once you have written your goal, you may begin to steer a course rather than drift aimlessly. Knowing where you want to go, before and during your journey, is important.

After you have a clearly defined written goal, you will find that making decisions is easier. If you know exactly where you want to go, it is a matter of deciding, "Yes, this will take me in the right direction" or "No, this will take me in the wrong direction."

To obtain great success or achievement, goals must take into consideration your unique individual qualities. Don't set yourself up for failure. Goals should be challenging, but attainable, based upon where you are starting and what you believe is possible for you.

Humans are goal-striving beings who find happiness in striving for and attaining worthwhile goals. Boredom is usually a result of not having goals. Some say that weight training is boring or that life is boring, but those who say this probably are not working toward worthwhile goals they are passionate about. If you know what you are trying to accomplish, weight training and life become exciting adventures — not easy, but certainly not boring. When people stop striving for goals, they stop growing.

Positive Thinking

Positive thinking is such an essential ingredient in success that some people have identified it as the *only* ingredient. One reason for this is that the goal-setting stage is primarily an internal process that others do not see. Positive thinking, by contrast, is obvious to everyone who comes in contact with the individual.

Your subconscious mind works on what you feed it. One sure way to short-circuit your success is to set a goal and not believe you can make it. Instead, you should fill your mind with positive thoughts, send out positive thoughts, and resist the negative thoughts of others. Positive people see the good side of bad situations and the bright side of every situation. Is a half glass of water half full or half empty? Your answer to that simple question may reveal a lot about your attitude. Many people dwell upon what they don't have and can't do; others focus upon what they do have and can do.

People should not strive for success without happiness. It would be an empty success even if the goal is achieved. Truly successful people enjoy what they are doing. Most people are as happy as they decide to be. Happiness is based on your internal reaction to external events.

Imagination is a stronger force than willpower. Form a clear, detailed image of what you really want. Everything starts with an idea. You will become that which you think about. If you dwell on failure, you will fail. If you dwell on success, you will succeed. Positive thoughts create positive things.

Desire is the power behind human action. Successful people have an all-consuming, burning desire to reach their goals.

Positive thinking includes belief. Belief is more than wishing; it is knowing that you can achieve your goal.

The Subconscious Mind

Nobody knows much about the subconscious mind, but we do know that it is extremely powerful and that it can help solve our problems. The subconscious mind works day and night to bring about what you imagine or visualize. That is why positive thinking is so important. If you think failure, you will fail. If you think success, you will succeed.

Your subconscious mind can be programmed through repetition. Repetition can accomplish great tasks. Therefore, you should read your goal aloud at least twice each day, morning and night, and read your weight training goal before each training session so you know why you are there and what you need to accomplish.

You have an opportunity to participate in your own creation. You can become what you want to become. You can be the person you want to be. To use your subconscious mind, use autosuggestion and repeat your desire or goal to yourself regularly. Once the idea is deeply embedded, the subconscious mind will go to work to help you achieve your goal. Keep a notepad and pencil handy for ideas; solutions will come to you. Write down these ideas immediately so you can expand on them later. Often, if they are not written down, they are gone. You may remember that you had a great idea but not be able to remember what it was.

A Written Plan

Everyone has the same amount of time each week. Why do some people accomplish more than others? They learn to manage themselves and use their time wisely. Lack of time indicates lack of organization. Some people say they don't have time to exercise. What they should say is that exercise is less important to them than anything else they do.

Effectiveness means doing the right things. This requires a focus on *result*s. Your time should be spent on the things that make a difference. In your weight training program, be sure you are doing the things that lead to achievement of your goal and do not waste your time on things that don't matter.

Efficiency means doing things right. This requires a focus on *methods*. Once you are doing the right exercises and you are doing the exercises right, you will be well on your way to reaching your goals.

Time should be planned to continue learning about weight training. The more you learn, the better you can plan to reach your goals.

Take time to plan how you will reach your goals, and continue to evaluate your progress toward your goals. After an evaluation, make the necessary adjustments in your plan.

Do It!

All of the previous steps are useless unless you take action. The world is controlled by people of action. You can never get anywhere unless you move. Therefore, decide what activities will lead to your goals, then act upon your decision. Learn to act and make things happen instead of merely reacting to things that happen to you.

Work and sacrifice are required to reach your goals. There is always a price to pay for anything that is worthwhile. You should not expect to get something for nothing. You must work at success. Once you have decided what must be done, discipline yourself to do it.

One of the most common reasons for failure is failure to take action. Procrastination has caused more failure than any other single factor. Now is the time to take action, not later, tomorrow, someday, or sometime. The clock is already running, and it cannot be stopped or reversed.

Once you get started, you must persist. Persistence is a familiar word but a rare quality. Many who take the first step fail because they do not continue working toward their goal. Stick with it, don't give up, never give up. If your goal is worthwhile, it is worth your best effort.

A formula for success that will work for almost anything you want is presented in this book to help you reach your weight training goals.

WRITING WEIGHT TRAINING GOALS

Your goals must be believable, achievable, reasonable, and attainable (Table 15.1). Don't set yourself up for failure. A goal to bench press 1,000 pounds by the end of this year is not reasonable. A goal to lose 20 pounds of fat by the end of the week is not possible. People should set goals that they can sincerely believe in. Once you reach a goal, you can always set a higher goal. Success breeds success.

Goals must be compatible. Running the marathon in under 2 hours and performing squats with 800 pounds on the same day are not compatible training goals.

Your weight training goals should be specific and measurable. Set a specific time for their attainment.

Complete the "Goal Setting" assignment at the end of this chapter. If you have too many goals, a conflict of interest may interfere with your progress. Rather than setting too many goals at one time, focus on a few things that are most important to you. If, however, you have several short-term body measurement goals that are compatible, and that lead to the same long-term goal of looking good,

STEPS IN THE FORMULA FOR SUCCESS

☑ Develop written goals.
- Set short-term goals that you can achieve that will lead to your long-term goals.
- Fix in your mind exact, measurable goals.
- Write down your goals.

☑ Use positive thinking.
- Believe you can reach your goals.
- Have faith in your ability to achieve your goals.

☑ Use your subconscious mind.
- Read your goals aloud at least twice each day, morning and night.
- Read your weight training goals before each training session.

☑ Develop a written plan.
- Take time to plan so that your efforts are directed toward your goals.
- Evaluate your progress and modify your plan.

☑ Do it.
- Start working toward your goal, and don't stop until you reach it.
- Enjoy the journey as much as the arrival.

you will be all right. The goals you set must be your own, not someone else's. They must be *your* goals, something *you* want.

If you do not want to increase your muscular strength, muscular size, or muscular endurance; if you do not want to perform better, look better, or feel better; if you cannot think of any goal that weight training can help you achieve — you probably will perceive weight training to be difficult, time-consuming, and boring. If you want to increase your muscular strength, muscular size, or muscular endurance; if you want to perform better, look better, or feel better; if you can think of a goal that weight training can help you achieve — you probably will perceive weight training to be worthwhile and interesting.

TABLE 15.1 Examples of Poor Goals and Good Goals

Poorly Written Goals	Well Written Goals
Increase my bench press. *(no set amount, no time limit)*	I will bench press 240 pounds one time by _____ *(day, month, year)*
Firm up my muscles. *(too general; how will you know?)*	I will perform 30 repetitions of the barbell curl using 60 pounds by _____ *(day, month, year)*
Get in shape. *(too general; how will you measure this?)*	I will have a 28-inch waist by _____ *(day, month, year)*

Name _____ Section _____

Goal Setting

Directions:

1. Read Chapter 15, A Formula for Success.

2. Make your weight training goals specific, measurable, believable, and compatible.

3. Set a specific date by which you will reach your goal.

4. Make the goals your goals, something you want very much. The greater your desire for the goal, the greater your chance of achieving it.

5. Include changes in muscular strength or size or endurance.

6. Write at least one, but not more than three, personal weight training goals. These should be short-term goals that can be reached in the next 3 months.

Goal 1: I will _____

_____

_____

by _____
                              (day, month, year)

Goal 2: I will _____

_____

_____

by _____
                              (day, month, year)

Goal 3: I will _____

_____

_____

by _____
                              (day, month, year)

Planning a Weight Training Program

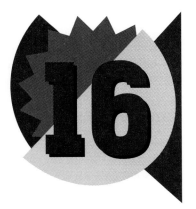

BASIC WEIGHT TRAINING PRINCIPLES

Three basic principles underlying all weight training progress are: specificity, overload, and progression.

Specificity

You must exercise the specific muscles that you want to develop. You also must follow specific exercise guidelines to produce the specific type of change you want to occur: muscle strength, muscle size, or muscle endurance.

Overload

The overload principle is the basis of all training programs. In weight training that means the muscle to be developed must be overloaded, or forced to work harder than normal.

Progression

Once your muscles adjust to a given workload, it no longer is an overload. The workload must be increased gradually as the muscle adapts to each new demand.

CONSIDERATIONS IN PLANNING YOUR WEIGHT TRAINING PROGRAM

Your Goals

Planning a weight training program must begin with what you wish to accomplish. You can train for three basic aspects of muscle fitness:

- Muscle strength.
- Muscle size.
- Muscle endurance.

Any weight training program you choose will result in some increase in all three areas. Untrained beginners gain on almost any weight training program as long as progressive overload is applied. Some general guidelines have emerged from research and experience that will help you focus on developing the aspect you are most interested in.

Which Exercises

Among the many weight training exercises to choose from, which ones are the best? The best weight training exercises are compound exercises, which require more than one joint or muscle to move the weight. With compound exercises, such as the squat and the bench press, large amounts of muscle are exercised at the same time. Exercises that require both arms or both legs to work together allow the use of more weight and maintain a balance of development on both sides of the body.

Almost all weight trainers use the same basic exercises. These exercises are included in the beginner or basic weight training program in this book.

Choose exercises for your training program with overall development in mind. Developing the entire body is better than ignoring certain body parts or overdeveloping one or two body parts. As you select your exercises, keep balanced development in mind. Both sides of the body should be developed equally, and the opposing muscle or muscle group should always be exercised. In the beginning, if you do not know the muscles, remember that for every exercise action or movement you perform, there should be an opposite action or movement in another exercise.

For example, if you perform an exercise that develops elbow flexion, you should also do an exercise that develops elbow extension.

Number of Exercises

One exercise per body part is enough for the beginning weight trainer. In fact, one exercise per body part is enough for all but the most advanced high-level strength athletes and body builders. For the first year or two of training, more than one exercise for each muscle group may result in overtraining and slow your progress. One exercise for each major muscle group or body part will result in about 8 to 12 basic exercises in your training program.

Order of Exercises

Exercise the largest muscles first and work your way down to the smallest muscles last. The largest muscles require the most energy and need the smaller muscles to assist. If the smaller muscles are already fatigued, you will have difficulty handling enough weight to properly exercise the larger muscles. For example, most back exercises require grip strength. If the finger and forearm flexors have already been exercised, they will fatigue before the larger back muscles. The largest muscles are located on the torso. Proceeding outward on the arms and legs, the muscles get smaller.

The order of exercises also may be based on a *work-rest principle*. If a muscle is worked during an exercise, it is allowed to rest during the next exercise. If you are exercising opposing muscle groups, you may work a muscle, then let it rest as you work on the opposing muscle. This allows you to complete more work in less time.

Another consideration in the order of exercises is whether to perform a circuit or to do the exercises in a traditional (non-circuit) manner. When you perform a circuit, you do each exercise in your training program once in a specified order. Then you perform each exercise again (and possibly again) in that same order. The traditional way of lifting weights is to do all of the sets of one exercise before moving to the next exercise.

Resistance

The amount of weight you use depends upon what you want to develop. The general rule is that for

strength you need a heavy weight and few repetitions. For muscle *endurance* you need a light weight and more repetitions. Muscle *size* development is in between, calling for moderate weight and repetitions. Before the heavy weight of strength training, you should complete warm-up sets.

Strength	85% to 100% of 1-RM
Muscle size	70% to 85% of 1-RM
Muscle endurance	50% to 70% of 1-RM

Starting Weight

Begin with a weight that is light so you can easily perform each exercise correctly. Increase the resistance gradually. Don't be in too big of a hurry to load up on resistance. If you give your body time to adapt, you will experience more progress, less muscle soreness, and less frustration. You have plenty of time to add weight if you are *Weight Training for Life*.

Repetitions

The resistance you choose will affect the repetitions you perform:

Strength	1–5 repetitions
Muscle size	6–12 repetitions
Muscle endurance	12–20+ repetitions

Most experienced weight trainers do moderate to high repetitions when they exercise the abdominals, lower back, forearms, and calves.

Sets

The resistance and repetitions influence the number of sets you will be able to perform for each exercise:

Strength	4–8 sets
Muscle size	3–6 sets
Muscle endurance	2–4 sets

Rest

The amount of rest between sets is determined by what you are trying to develop:

Strength	2–4 minutes
Muscle size	1–2 minutes
Muscle endurance	30–90 seconds

TABLE 16.1 Summary of Weight Training Guidelines

	Muscle Strength	Muscle Size	Muscle Endurance	Muscle Tone
Resistance	85% to 100% of 1-RM	70% to 85% of 1-RM	50% to 70% of 1-RM	60% to 80% of 1-RM
Repetitions	1 to 6 RM	6 to 12 RM	12 to 20 + RM	8 to 12 RM
Sets	4 to 8	3 to 6	2 to 4	1 to 3
Rest (between sets)	2 to 4 minutes	1 to 2 minutes	30 to 90 seconds	30 to 60 seconds

Frequency

A muscle usually requires 2 or 3 days of rest to recover and adapt before it should be exercised again. Exercising a muscle 3 days per week with 48 to 72 hours of rest between training sessions works well for most weight trainers. Advanced weight trainers perform different exercises on different days, so they may exercise 4, 5, or 6 days a week; they do not exercise the same body parts each day.

Fixed or Variable Exercise Load

A load is applied to each exercise in two basic ways: fixed or variable. With a *fixed load* the resistance, repetitions, sets, and rest interval remain the same (fixed) during a training session for an exercise.

Example: Bench Press
        150 pounds
         10 repetitions
         3 sets
         1 minute rest between sets

With a *variable method* of loading, the resistance, repetitions, and rest interval change for each set of an exercise.

Example: Bench Press
        150 lbs 10 reps 1 min. rest
        170 lbs 8 reps 2 min. rest
        190 lbs 6 reps 3 min. rest
        210 lbs 4 reps 4 min. rest

Progression

Some general rules will be helpful in applying the progression principle to the overload:

- Increase only one variable at a time (resistance, repetitions, sets, rest).
- Increase reps or sets before increasing resistance.
- Decrease reps when increasing resistance.
- Decrease the rest interval between sets to increase muscular endurance.

Muscle Tone or Muscle Fitness

Beginners often say they just want to tone the muscles. They are not especially interested in developing strength, size, or endurance.

What is muscle tone? When the word "tone" is used in reference to muscle tissue, it refers to muscle tissue that is firm, sound, and resilient. This is in contrast to the loose, flabby, and weak muscle tone of the sedentary person. Although the former is desirable, measuring changes in muscle tone is rather difficult.

Whether a person chooses to train for strength, size, or endurance, an improvement in muscle tone will occur. Also, if an individual chooses to train for muscle tone, some improvement will occur in strength, size, and muscle endurance. These improvements, however, will be more gradual and more difficult to measure.

Some guidelines for those who wish to train for muscle fitness or muscle tone are:

    60% to 80% of 1-RM
    8 to 12 repetitions
    1 to 3 sets of each exercise
    30 to 60 seconds rest between sets
    3 days per week (every other day)

Although training for muscle tone is possible, the lack of measurable progress can result in a loss of motivation for beginners. Therefore, beginning weight trainers are advised to work toward changes in strength, size, or muscle endurance, which can be measured more easily. Measured progress is evidence that weight training is effective, and it serves as a motivating influence to continue.

SUGGESTED LIFETIME FITNESS WEIGHT TRAINING PROGRAMS

The following training programs are appropriate for adults as lifetime weight training programs

1×15–20
1×8–12
2×10
3×10
3×8
$3 \times 10, 8, 6$
$3 \times 20, 10, 5$
DeLorme 3×10

The 1×15-20 workout is one in which you perform one set of each exercise, attempting to complete 20 repetitions. If you complete all 20 repetitions in good exercise form, the weight on that exercise can be increased for the next training session. You always should be able to complete at least 15 good repetitions. If you cannot complete at least 15 repetitions, the weight is too heavy. If you can complete more than 20 repetitions, the weight is too light.

The 1×8-12 workout is the same as the previous workout except that you should be able to get at least 8 repetitions and you should raise the weight if you can get more than 12 good strict repetitions. This and the previous workout are two fast weight training programs for those who do not want to spend much time weight training.

The 2×10, 3×10, and 3×8 workouts can be performed using the same weight for two or three sets with a short 1- or 2-minute rest between sets. If you are able to complete all of the repetitions in every set, the weight can be increased for the next training session.

The $3 \times 10, 8,$ and 6 workout consists of three sets. The first set calls for 10 repetitions, the second set, 8 repetitions. In the third set you perform 6 repetitions. Each set is done with a heavier weight.

The (3×20, 10, 5 workout includes three sets of each exercise. The first set calls for 20 repetitions. Twenty repetitions will provide a good warm up as well as a stimulus for developing muscle endurance. The second set calls for 10 repetitions. Ten repetitions will provide some stimulus for muscle endurance gain, some stimulus for muscle size gain, and some stimulus for strength gain. The third set calls for 5 repetitions. The first two sets should have the muscles and joints warmed up and ready for this heavier load. Five repetitions with a heavy resistance will provide a stimulus for strength gain.

The DeLorme 3×10 workout consists of three sets of 10 repetitions:

1st set:	10 reps with	50% of 10 RM
2nd set:	10 reps with	75% of 10 RM
3rd set:	10 reps with	100% of 10 RM

The first set of 10 repetitions should be performed with 50% of your 10 repetition maximum (10-RM). Your 10-repetition maximum is the heaviest weight you can lift 10 times. The second set of 10 repetitions should be performed with 75% of your 10-repetition maximum. The third set should be performed with 100% of your 10-repetition maximum.

When you can complete 10 repetitions in the third set, the weight used in that set is raised for the next training session and the first two sets are adjusted according to this new 10-RM. You should be able to get about 8 repetitions in the last set with the new weight. Keep working with that weight until you can get 10 good repetitions. Then the weight is raised again. You should never get fewer than 6 good repetitions in the last set. If you cannot get at least 6 good repetitions, you have increased the weight too much and should reduce the weight for the next training session.

The DeLorme method is fast and easy on weight-stack machines but involves quite a bit of weight changing when using barbells, especially when alternating sets with a training partner.

Based on the information presented in this chapter, complete "Planning Your Personal Weight Training Program" using the chart provided in the at the end of this chapter.

Name _____ Section _____

Planning Your Personal Weight Training Program

Directions:

1. Read Chapter 16, Planning a Weight Training Program.
2. Plan an exercise program that is consistent with your goals.
3. Refer to the Exercise chapters for general body part and specific exercises.
4. Refer to Chapter 16 for resistance, repetitions, sets, rest, and frequency.

General Body Part	Specific Exercise	Resistance % of 1-RM	Repetitions	Sets	Rest Interval	Frequency Days/wk.

Name _____   Section _____

Date													
Exercise	Wt	Rep	Wt	Rep	Wt	Rep	Wt	Rep	Wt	Rep	Wt	Rep

Name _____ Section _____

Date													
Exercise	Wt	Rep	Wt	Rep	Wt	Rep	Wt	Rep	Wt	Rep	Wt	Rep

Name _____ Section _____

Date												
Exercise	Wt	Rep	Wt	Rep	Wt	Rep	Wt	Rep	Wt	Rep	Wt	Rep

Name _____   Section _____

Date													
Exercise	Wt	Rep	Wt	Rep	Wt	Rep	Wt	Rep	Wt	Rep	Wt	Rep

Advanced Weight Training

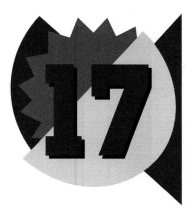

PROGRESSIVE OVERLOAD

Progressive overload is the basis of all successful weight training programs. The muscles can be overloaded in many ways. The overload that the muscles experience depends upon all of the following variables:

- Which exercises are performed.
- How many total exercises are performed.
- How many exercises are performed for each body part.
- Order in which exercises are performed.
- Amount of resistance or weight used in each set.
- Number of repetitions per set.
- Number of sets per exercise.
- Amount of rest between sets.
- Frequency of training sessions.
- Method of progression.
- Whether the exercise load is fixed or variable.
- Whether the total body is exercised in each training session or is divided into a split routine.
- Exercise intensity.

These variables may be changed and combined in a seemingly unlimited number of ways. Some of the more common training programs will be presented to give you an idea of the variety available to you in weight training. All of these training programs are different ways to arrive at the same thing: progressive overload.

Beginning weight trainers tend to gain on almost any weight training program. The greatest danger for beginners is overtraining. If you find yourself training very hard, not making any progress, and feeling tired all the time, you probably are overtraining and should try less exercise and more rest.

Humans cannot maintain absolute peak condition for very long — probably a few weeks at best. Therefore, highly trained advanced weight trainers, competitive lifters, and body builders use periodization or cycling. They divide the year into periods or cycles, then vary their training methods and intensity during the cycles so they reach their peak condition during their competitive season, and hopefully for their most important contest of the year.

INCREASING EXERCISE INTENSITY

One of the first things that weight trainers try to do as they advance in their training is to increase the intensity of their exercise. The following are seven common methods of increasing exercise intensity. All these methods increase your risk of injury. Be very careful.

Concentric Failure

To reach concentric failure, you must perform repetitions until you cannot perform another repetition while maintaining strict exercise form.

Forced Reps

Forced reps are repetitions performed after reaching concentric failure. When you cannot perform another repetition correctly by yourself, a spotter assists as little as possible to help you complete one or two more repetitions.

153

Negatives

You can lower a heavier weight than you can lift. Negatives are performed by having spotters help you lift a weight and then allowing you to lower the weight by yourself. This is an advanced training method that can result in extreme muscle soreness. It is not recommended for beginning weight trainers.

Eccentric Failure

When you perform negatives (lower a weight) until you can no longer control the speed at which you lower the weight, you have reached eccentric failure. This is obviously dangerous and is not recommended.

Cheating

Cheating is the use of body movement to get past the weakest point in the range of motion of an exercise. It can be a useful means for advanced lifters to add to the overload; however, most weight trainers cheat to make the exercise easier.

Pre-Exhaustion

Pre-exhaustion involves performing an isolation exercise for a muscle and following this immediately by a compound exercise. The idea is to work the muscle to concentric failure with the isolation exercise, then to force the muscle to continue working with the assistance of other muscles that are not exhausted.

Cycle or Periodization

Advanced lifters use training cycles or periods in which they vary exercise intensity and volume to reach a peak during their competitive season.

Beginning weight trainers do not need to use any of these methods of increasing exercise intensity as long as they are making steady progress.

TOTAL BODY AND SPLIT ROUTINES

Total Body Training Routines

Beginners and fitness weight trainers often perform all of their weight training exercises at one time and repeat this procedure every other day. They exercise the total body in one training session.

Split Routines

As weight trainers advance and the total workload increases, many choose to split their exercises, performing part of them one day and the rest of them on another day. One example is the 4-day split, in which half of the exercises are performed on Monday and Thursday and the other half on Tuesday and Friday. An example of a 4-day split is a push-pull routine in which the pushing exercises are performed on Monday and Thursday and the pulling exercises on Tuesday and Friday.

Many advanced body builders go to a 6-day split as they near competition. In a 6-day split they perform about a third of their exercises on Monday and Thursday, a third on Tuesday and Friday, and a third on Wednesday and Saturday. The ultimate split is the blitz routine, in which they exercise only one body part each day.

FIXED SYSTEMS

Fixed systems are those in which variables are not changed during a training session but a variable may be changed for the next training session.

Simple Progressive System

A simple progressive system involves changing only one variable, such as the resistance. An example is performing one set of 10 repetitions of an exercise. If 10 repetitions are completed, the weight is increased for the next training session.

Double Progressive System

A double progressive system calls for changing two variables, such as resistance and repetitions. An example is performing one set of 12 repetitions. If 12 repetitions are completed, the weight is increased for the next training session and the repetitions are decreased to 8. The repetitions then are increased by one each training session until one set of 12 repetitions is completed with the new weight. Then the weight is increased and the repetitions are decreased again. This pattern continues — increasing the repetitions, then the weight.

One Set to Failure

A variation of the double progressive system is one set to failure. In this system one set of each exercise is performed to the point at which you cannot perform another repetition and still maintain correct exercise form. A weight is used that causes this failure to occur between 8 and 12 repetitions. When you complete 12 repetitions, the weight is increased for the next training session.

Set System

The set system requires the lifter to perform more than one set of each exercise. In a fixed system the repetitions remain the same for each set. One example is three sets of 6 repetitions. When you can perform 6 repetitions in all three sets, the weight is raised for the next training session. This is a good program if you are training with barbells because it reduces the amount of time you spend changing weights.

Circuit System

A series of exercises is performed in a sequence or circuit with one exercise at each station. You move from one exercise to the next, performing one set of each exercise until you have completed every exercise in the circuit once. The entire circuit then may be repeated. A circuit usually is completed one to three times during a training session.

Circuit training often is used with a large group when time and equipment are limited. This is often the case with athletic teams. Circuit training allows a large number of people to get a good workout in a short time.

Aerobic Circuit System

In an aerobic weight training circuit, exercises are performed one right after the other with very little rest between exercises. This is done to keep the heart rate elevated during the entire circuit and thus produce a training effect for the cardiovascular system.

Super Set System

A super set requires performing two exercises in a sequence, followed by a rest interval. Often, opposing muscle groups are exercised in this manner. For example, the first set might consist of barbell curls

for the elbow flexors. The next exercise could be tricep extensions for the elbow extensors. Because these muscles work in opposition to one another, one of them is resting while the other is working. After one set of each exercise, there is usually a rest interval before repeating the sequence. This is a good way to reduce training time without reducing the amount of work completed during the training session. It is like a mini-circuit.

Giant Sets

Giant sets usually involve three to five exercises for the same muscle. One set of each exercise is performed with little or no rest between sets. After all of the exercises in the sequence have been performed, there is a rest interval before the sequence is repeated. This is a highly advanced training system that some body builders use.

Rest-Pause System

The rest-pause system has many variations. Here is one: Perform an exercise to the point of temporary muscular failure, hold the weight while the muscle recovers slightly, perform another repetition, pause, do another repetition, continue until no more repetitions can be performed.

VARIABLE SYSTEMS

In variable systems one or more variables are altered during the performance of one exercise.

Pyramid System

In a pyramid system the weight used for each set of an exercise is increased and the number of repetitions is decreased correspondingly. This allows the exerciser to proceed from a light weight to a heavy weight. This system is used most often by those training for strength. Some choose to pyramid up only; others pyramid up to a heavy weight, then back down again.

Percentage System

This is a variation of the pyramid system. Multiple sets of an exercise are performed at various percentages of the 1-RM for that exercise. The percentages usually start out low in the first set and increase in each of the subsequent sets.

DeLorme System

One good percentage system for beginners, and those training for fitness, is the DeLorme system:

1st set	10 reps	50% of 10-RM
2nd set	10 reps	75% of 10-RM
3rd set	10 reps	100% of 10-RM

Continuous Set System

In the continuous set system you start with a weight that you can use to complete a given number of repetitions — for example, 10 repetitions. When you reach the point at which you can do no more repetitions, your training partner quickly removes a small amount of weight while you continue to hold the bar or stay in position on the machine. As soon as some weight has been removed, the exercise is continued until you cannot do any more repetitions. Once again, your training partner removes a small amount of weight. This process continues until you cannot do any more repetitions, even with the lightest weight.

Light to Heavy System

In this variation of the pyramid and continuous set systems, you start with a light to moderate weight and perform 3 repetitions. Your training partners quickly add a small amount of weight. After 3 more repetitions you again add weight. This process continues until you can perform only one repetition.

Tonnage System

The resistance and repetitions vary in the tonnage system, but the lifter keeps track of the total pounds lifted in a training session. This is used most often by competitive weight lifters.

These are only a few of the methods that advanced weight trainers have used to improve their training progress. Many more are in use.

TRAINING EQUIPMENT

Constant External Resistance Equipment

Barbells, dumbbells, and some weight-stack equipment have a resistance that is constant. The weight remains the same throughout the exercise. Because of changes in leverage at the joints involved during movement through the full range of motion, this fixed weight is more difficult to lift at some joint angles and easier at others.

With constant external resistance equipment you are limited to the heaviest weight you can lift through the weakest point in the range of motion. Two basic equipment design approaches have attempted to overcome this limitation: variable resistance equipment and isokinetic equipment.

Variable Resistance Equipment

Some weight-stack equipment has been designed so that as changes in leverage take place for the working muscles and joints, the exercise machine makes compensating leverage changes. When you are exercising with constant external resistance equipment, once you can get past the weakest point in the range of motion, the rest of the exercise movement is fairly easy. With the compensating leverage change of variable resistance equipment, the muscle must continue to work hard throughout the full range of motion.

The weight in the stack lifted remains constant, but the leverage change in the machine makes the resistance greater at some joint angles and less at other joint angles. The intent of variable resistance equipment is to keep the muscles fully loaded throughout the full range of motion.

Isokinetic Equipment

Isokinetic equipment offers another solution to keeping the muscle fully loaded throughout the full range of motion. Isokinetic refers to constant motion or constant speed. True isokinetic exercise equipment limits the speed at which the exercise device will move. Therefore, a muscle can contract at its maximum force from full extension to full contraction without producing acceleration.

Which Type of Exercise Equipment is the Best?

So far, no one particular type of exercise equipment has been proven superior for the development of muscle tissue. Muscles don't know or care what type of exercise equipment is used to provide the resistance as long as they receive the same overload stimulus.

Tips for Sticking With It

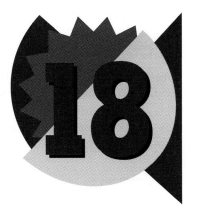

Anyone can start a weight training program, and many do, but few will stick with it. The following are some tips for sticking with your weight training program and getting the results you want.

MOTIVATION

Unmet needs and wants motivate your behavior. The depth of your desire to meet that need or want determines the strength of your motivation. Once you reach your goal it loses its power to motivate. After all, now you have what you wanted. To get the motivation to continue weight training you need to set a new goal. The new goal could be further improvement or it could be maintenance of what you have achieved.

ENJOYMENT

Enjoyment is extremely important to sticking with your weight training program. Most normal people seek pleasure and avoid pain. Most people find time for the activities they enjoy and find excuses to avoid the activities that are difficult and painful for them. If you enjoy weight training, then you will find a way to do it on a regular basis. If you design a personal weight training program for yourself that is a long, boring, terrible, painful experience, then you will find excuses to avoid it. Different people find exercise enjoyment, or satisfaction, in different ways. Some of the things that bring weight training enjoyment include improvement, challenge, excitement, relaxation, competition, and social interaction.

IMPORTANCE

Regular, lifelong weight trainers have a common belief that weight training is good for them. There is a lot of evidence to support that belief. If you haven't read the evidence yet, maybe you should start now. To continue regular weight training you must believe that the benefits you receive from your program are worth the time, effort, energy, and money you put into it.

PRIORITY

To stick with it you must place a high priority on your weight training program. Build it into your schedule and stick with the time you have set for training. There will always be other things you could do during that time, but don't allow those other things to replace your training time.

TIME

We all have the same amount of time each year, each month, each week, and each day. Some people make time for exercise and some claim they don't have time to exercise. Surveys have indicated that the average American watches three to four hours of television each day, and yet these same people claim they do not have time to exercise. Clearly, for most people it is not a question of time, but one of priorities. Schedule your weight training time and stick with it.

RECORD

Improvement is a powerful motivator for most people. Write down the relevant information from each weight training session. These records will provide visible evidence of your improvement and of your ability to stick with a weight training program.

REWARD

Regular weight trainers generally get a sense of satisfaction, an intrinsic reward, from regular exercise sessions. However, as a beginner you may benefit from extrinsic rewards. You might want to promise yourself something for reaching a goal you have set for yourself. Of course, it should be a healthy reward and you should only get it if you reach your goal.

LEARN

The more you learn about weight training, the more you understand the benefits, the more you know about correct technique, the more you know about designing programs, the more likely you are to continue. Most people want to be good at something. If you are willing to study, and stick with your training, you can become good at weight training.

SOCIAL

Some people enjoy the social aspects of weight training. They enjoy exercising with a friend or a small group. They enjoy the new friends they meet when they are weight training. If you meet people while you are weight training, you instantly have something in common, and a topic of conversation, with them.

SUPPORT

Share your new weight training goals and your new weight training program with people you know will be supportive. Get support from as many people as you can. Once you tell a large number of people you are going to do something it becomes harder to quit and easier to continue.

IDENTITY

Once you become a regular weight trainer it becomes a part of your identity. Once it is a part of who you are and what you do, it is easier to stick with it and harder to quit. Friends and family no longer ask if you are going to workout, instead they ask when you are going to workout.

PLACE

Find or create a pleasant place to do your weight training. If you like the place where you exercise, you will want to go there. If you don't like the place where you do your weight training you will not want to go there.

CONVENIENCE

If weight training is too inconvenient you are more likely to quit. Find ways to make weight training as convenient as possible. Identify the obstacles to regular weight training and, one by one, begin to eliminate them.

INSTRUCTION

Most people get satisfaction from doing something well. Getting good instruction whenever you start a new activity is usually an excellent investment of your time and money. Excellent instruction gets you past the awkward beginner stage more quickly. Weight training is no exception. Getting good weight training instruction when you are beginning will get you past the beginner stage more quickly and will help you avoid mistakes.

VARIETY

There is a great deal of variation when it comes to variety in your weight training program. Some people prefer a very structured routine that almost never changes. They like to do the same exercises in the same order at the same time on the same days for years. Others like to do something different every training session. Most people are somewhere in between. They like to follow an exercise plan for 6 weeks or 8 weeks or 12 weeks or some other block of time, then change their program for the next block of time. You need to determine what works best for you, what keeps the training fun and interesting for you.

CHAPTER 18

FITNESS

If you can stick with a weight training program long enough to reach a fitness level you are proud of, you are more likely to continue to train for the rest of your life. It is much easier to maintain a higher level of fitness than it is to get there in the first place.

SUCCESS

You can learn to set reasonable goals. You can learn to plan weight training programs to reach your goals. You can learn to stick with your weight training program. You can improve your fitness level. You can achieve success through weight training.

APPEARANCE

In our society appearance is important. We are bombarded by constant daily messages that looking good is important. Movies, television, and advertising continually stress the importance of looking good. It is ok to want to improve your appearance and look good. While having a good body is attractive, self-worship is not attractive. One of the most effective and efficient ways to improve your appearance is weight training.

IMAGE

Everyone has a body image. Your body image is how you see yourself. Most people have a subconscious drive to maintain a body that is consistent with their body image. In other words, those who see themselves as fit make lifestyle choices that keep them fit.

A perfect body is not possible, even if we could come to some general worldwide total agreement of what the perfect body would look like. Training for perfection is unrealistic and unattainable. Instead train for a healthy body image. You can not change your genetic body type, but you can make the most of what you have.

REGULARITY

The greatest benefits of weight training come from a lifelong habit of regular training. The winners are those who have perseverance and are consistent in their training. The losers will go at weight training too hard for a short time, then quit and do nothing for a long time. They may start again, but they generally go too hard again for a short time, then quit again. By contrast, the winners generally have a more moderate pace and more realistic weight training programs. They design weight training programs they can stick with for years. Good habits bring good results.

HABIT

The body adapts gradually to weight training. Faster in the beginning and slower as you progress. Healthy weight training is a healthy lifestyle habit much like brushing your teeth. It is most effective if it is done on a regular basis throughout your life.

SIMPLE HOME TRAINING PROGRAM FOR BUSY PEOPLE

This is a simple training program you can do at home. It takes very little time and very little money, but it can make a very big difference. The only equipment required is a set of two adjustable-weight dumbbells and a flat exercise bench. You can often find these items very inexpensively at garage sales. The 8 exercises are as follows:

Chest	Dumbbell Bench Press
Back	One-Dumbbell Rowing
Shoulders	Seated Dumbbell Lateral Raise
Arms (Biceps)	Seated Dumbbell Arm Curls
Arms (Triceps)	Seated One-Dumbbell Triceps Extension
Hips and Thighs	Dumbbell Lunges
Lower Leg	One-Dumbbell Calf Raise
Abdominals	Crunches

Perform these exercises every other day. If it takes one minute to perform each exercise and one minute between exercises, to rest and change the weight for the next exercise, you would complete this workout in 16 minutes. Realistically, plan on 20 minutes, especially as the resistance increases. For better total fitness results, perform 20 minutes of continuous aerobic exercise on non-lifting days. Convenient, inexpensive aerobic exercises include walking, jogging, and stair-stepping at home.

If this is still too time consuming split the weight-training program performing the upper body exercises one day (the first five exercises) and the lower body exercises the next day (the last three exercises). The upper body workout would take approximately 10 minutes every other day and the lower body workout would take about 6 minutes every other day.

During the first month perform one set of 20 repetitions of each exercise. The second month perform one set of 15 repetitions of each exercise. The third month perform one set of 12 repetitions of each exercise. After three months you may want to just maintain on this workout or you may want to try some of the other set and repetition combinations suggested in Chapter 16.

WEIGHT TRAINING FOR LIFE

If you don't take care of your body where will you live? Do you know people who take better care of their house or their car than their body? You may live in many houses and own many cars in your lifetime, but you only get this one body to live in for your entire life. Take good care of it by *weight training for life.*

Dumbbell Bench Press
(see page 42)

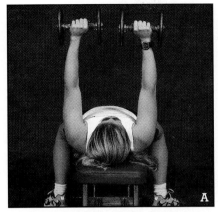

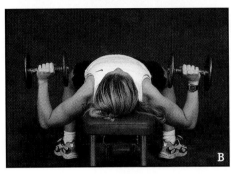

One-Dumbbell Rowing
(see page 52)

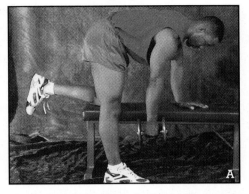

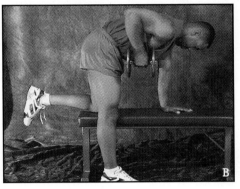

Dumbbell
Lateral Raise
(see page 64)

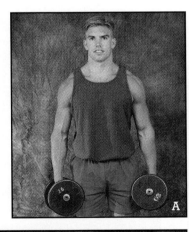

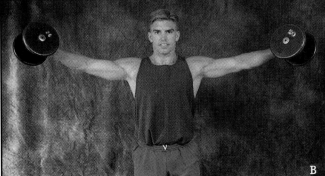

Seated Dumbbell Arm Curl
(see page 70)

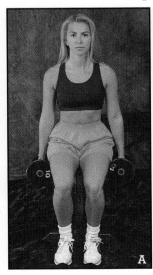

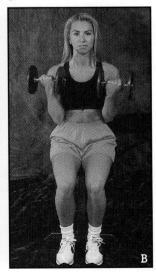

Seated One-Dumbbell Triceps Extension
(see page 74)

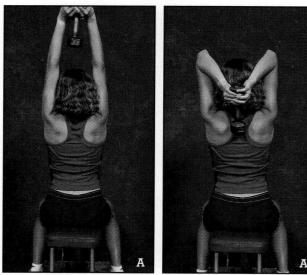

Dumbbell Lunges
(see page 88)

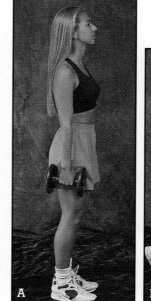
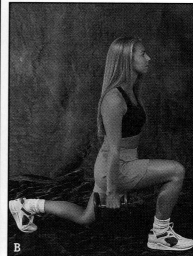

One-Dumbbell Calf Raise
(see page 96)

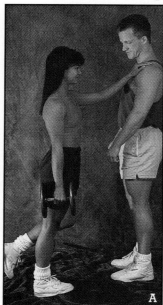
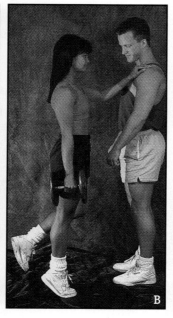

Crunches
(see page 100)

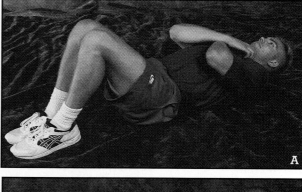
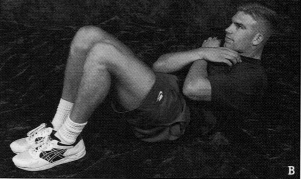

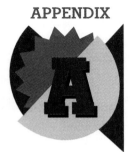

Internet Sites

American Alliance for Health, Physical Education, Recreation, and Dance (AAHPERD)
http://www.aahperd.org

American College of Sports Medicine (ACSM)
http://www.acsm.org/sportsmed

American Dietetics Association
http://www.eatright.org

American Running and Fitness Association
http://www.arfa.org

American Heart Association
http://www.amhrt.org

American Medical Association
http://www.ama-assn.org

Ask the Dietitian
http://www.hoptechno.com/rdindex.htm

Bodybuilding
http://www.bodyforlife.com/

Bodybuilding
http://www.muscle-fitness.com

Center for Disease Control and Prevention
http://www.cdc.gov

Center for Science in the Public Interest
http://www.cspinet.org

CNN's Health Report
http://www.cnn.com/Health

Diet Analysis Web Page
http://dawp.futuresouth.com/

Dr. Koop's Community
http://www.drkoop.com

Duke University Diet and Fitness Center Home Page
http://dmi-www.mc.duke.edu/dfc/home.html

Fast Food Finder
http://www.olen.com/food/

FDA Center for Food Safety and Applied Nutrition
http://vm.cfsan.fda.gov/list.html

FitnessLinks to the Internet
http://www.fitnesslink.com/links.htm

Fitness World
http://www.fitnessworld.com

Food and Nutrition Center of the
U.S. Department of Agriculture
http://www.nal.usda.gov/fnic

General Nutrition Site
http://www.healthy.net/index.html

Health A to Z
http://www.HealthAtoZ.com

Healthfinder
http://www.healthfinder.gov

Healthy People 2000
http://odphp.osophs.dhhs.gov/pubs/hp2000/

Mayo Clinic Health Information
http://www.mayo.ivi.com

Meals Online
http://www/meals.com

Medscape
http://www.medscape.com

National Bodybuilding and Fitness Magazine
http://nbaf.com/nbaf/hom.html

National Health Information Center (NHIC)
http://nhic-nt.health.org/

National Institutes of Health
http://www.nih.gov/health/

Nutrition Sites on the Internet
http://wce.uwyo.edu/wctl/high/nutr/default.html

Olympic Lifting
http://www.lifttilyadie.com

Olympic Lifting
http://www.goheavy.com/olympic

Pointer to Frequently asked Questions
about Weight Lifting
http://www.imp.mtu.edu/~babucher/weights/pointer.
html#FAQs

Power Lifting
http://www.powerlifting.com

Power Lifting
http://www.drsquat.com/

President's Council on Physical Fitness and Sports
http://www.hoptechno.com/book11.htm

Shape Up America!
http://www.shapeup.org

Stanford Health Link
http://healthlink.stanford.edu/

Stretching Information
http://www.enteract.com/~bradapp/docs/rec/
stretching_1.html

The Fitness Partner Connection Jumpsite
http://www.primusweb.com/fitnesspartner/

The Internet's Fitness Resource
http://rampages.onramp.net/~chaz/

The Physical Activity and Health Network (PAHNet)
http://www.pitt.edu/~pahnet/

The Powerlifting Competition —
Frequently asked Questions
http://www.cs.unc.edu/~wilsonk/power.faq.html

USA Weightlifting
http://www.usaw.org-usa

USDA Food and Nutrition Information Center
http://www.nalusda.gov/fnic/

United States Olympic Committee Sports from A to Z
http://www.olympic-usa.org/sports/

Virtual Vegetarian
http://www.vegetariantimes.com/

Weight Lifting: Olympic Style
http://www.waf.com/weights/index.htm

Welcome to The National Strength
and Conditioning Association
http://www.colosoft.com/nsca/

Worldguide Forum on Health and Fitness
http://www.worldguide.com/Fitness/hf.html

Yahoo Health Directory
http://www.yahoo.com/health

References and Suggested Readings

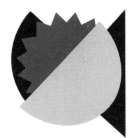

Aaberg, E. *Resistance Training Instruction*. Champaign, IL: Human Kinetics, 1999.

ACSM "The Recommended Quantity and Quality of Exercise for Developing and Maintaining Cardiovascular and Muscular Fitness, and Flexibility in Healthy Adults" *Med. Sci. Sports Exerc.*, Vol. 30. No. 6. Pp. 975-991, 1998.

ACSM "Exercise and Physical Activity for Older Adults" *Med.Sci. Sports, Exerc.*, Vol. 30. No. 6. Pp. 992-1008. 1998.

Allsen, P. E. *Strength Training: Beginners, Bodybuilders, and Athletes* (2nd edition). Dubuque, IA: Kendall/Hunt Publishing Company, 1996.

Alter, M. J. *Sport Stretch* (2nd edition). Champaign, IL: Human Kinetics, 1998.

Anderson, B., Burke, E., and Pearl, B. *Getting in Shape*. Bolinas, CA: Shelter Publications, Inc. 1994.

Baechle, T. R. *Essentials of Strength Training and Conditioning*. Champaign, IL: Human Kinetics, 1994.

Baechle, T. R. and Earle, R. W. *Fitness Weight Training*. Champaign, IL: Human Kinetics, 1995.

Baechle, T. R. and Groves, B. R. *Weight Training: Steps to Success* (2nd edition). Champaign, IL: Human Kinetics, 1998.

Bennett, J. *The Basics of Weight Training Workbook*. Boston, MA: Allyn and Bacon, 1995.

Brzycki, M. *A Practical Approach to Strength Training* (3rd edition) Indianapolis, IN; Masters Press, 1995.

Daniel, E. L. *Jump Start With WebLinks: A Guidebook for Fitness/Wellness/Personal Health*. Englewood, CO: Morton Publishing Company, 1997.

Fahey, T. *Basic Weight Training for Men and Women* (3nd edition). Mountain View, CA: Mayfield Publishing Company, 1997.

Fahey, T. D. and Hutchinson, G. *Weight Training for Women*. Mountain View, CA: Mayfield Publishing Company, 1992.

Field, R. W. and Roberts, S. O. *Weight Training*. Boston, MA: WCB/McGraw-Hill, 1999.

Fleck, S. J. and Kraemer, W. J. *Designing Resistance Training Programs* (2nd edition). Champaign, IL: Human Kinetics, 1997.

Grant, N. G. *Resistive Weight Training* (2nd edition). Dubuque, IA: Kendall/Hunt Publishing Company, 1993.

Hoeger, W. W. K. *Lifetime Physical Fitness and Wellness* (5th edition). Englewood, CO: Morton Publishing Company, 1998.

Hoeger, W. W. K. and Hoeger, S. A. *Principles and Labs for Fitness and Wellness* (5th edition). Englewood, CO: Morton Publishing Company, 1999.

Howley, E. T. and Franks, B. D. *Health Fitness Instructor's Handbook* (3rd edition). Champaign, IL: Human Kinetics, 1997.

Kraemer, W. J. and Fleck, S. J. *Strength Training for Young Athletes*. Champaign, IL: Human Kinetics Publishers, 1993.

Kubik, B. D. *Dinosaur Training: Lost Secrets of Strength and Development*. Louisville, KY, 1996

Mills, B. D. and Mitchell, C. A. *Jump Start With WebLinks: A Guidebook for Sport Education and Activities.* Englewood, CO: Morton Publishing Company, 1997.

NSCA Certification Commission. *Exercise Technique Checklist Manual*. Lincoln, NE: NSCA Certification Commission, 1997.

O'Connor, C. *Beginning Weight Training*. Boston, MA: American Press, 1993.

Peterson, J. A., Bryant, C. X., and Peterson, S. L. *Strength Training for Women*. Champaign, IL: Human Kinetics, 1995.

Rasch, P. J. *Weight Training* (5th edition). Dubuque, IA: Wm. C. Brown Publishers, 1990.

Roberts, S. O. and Pillarella, D. *Developing Strength in Children: A Comprehensive Guide*. Reston, VA: The American Alliance for Health, Physical Education, Recreation, and Dance, 1996.

Seidler, T. L., Waters, D. L., and Wilson, W. L. *Weight Training and Fitness for Health and Performance*. Dubuque, IA; Kendall/Hunt Publishing Company, 1990.

Seiger, L. H., Kanipe, E., Vanderpool, K., and Barnes, D. *Fitness and Wellness Strategies* (2nd edition). Boston, MA: WCB/McGraw-Hill, 1998.

Seiger, L. H. and Hesson, J. L. *Walking for Fitness* (2nd edition). Dubuque, IA: WCB/Brown and Benchmark Publishers, 1994.

Signorile, J. F., Tuten, R., Moore, C., and Knight, V. *Weight Training Everyone* (4th edition). Winston-Salem, NC; Hunter Textbooks, Inc., 1993.

Silvester, L. J. *Weight Training for Strength and Fitness*. Boston, MA: Jones and Bartlett Publishers, 1992.

Trestrail, R. T., *Weight Training: A Practical Approach to Total Fitness*. Dubuque, IA: Kendall/Hunt Publishing Company, 1994.

WCB/McGraw-Hill. *Health Net: A Health and Wellness Guide to The Internet*. Boston, MA: WCB/McGraw-Hill, 1999.

Westcott, W. *Be Strong: Strength Training for Muscular Fitness for Men and Women*. Dubuque, IA: Wm. C. Brown, Inc., 1993.

Westcott, W. L. and Baechle, T. R. *Strength Training Past 50*. Champaign, IL: Human Kinetics, 1998.

Index

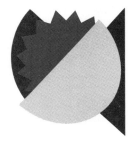

Ab Solution, 108
Abdominal crunch
  Nautilus machine, 101
Abdominal exercises
  crunches, 100
  curl-ups, 100
  Cybex abdominal machine, 101
  hanging knee raises, 105
  Nautilus abdominal machine, 101
  reverse crunches, 103
  seated reverse crunches, 104
  sit-ups, 102
  tuck-ups, 103
Abdominal obliques, 100–105
Actin, 13
Aerobic exercise, 116
Alcohol, 118
All-or-none Principle, 14
American Heart Association, 112
Amino acids, 113
Ankle plantar flexion
  calf press on Cybex leg press, 97
  one-dumbbell calf raise, 96
  seated calf raise, 97
  standing barbell calf raise, 94
  standing calf raise, machine, 95
  standing dumbbell calf raise, 96
  Universal heel raise, 95
Anterior deltoid, 42–47, 76–79
Arm curl
  Nautilus machine, 71
  Universal machine, 71
Arm exercises
  barbell curl, 14, 70
  barbell wrist curl, 80
  bench dips, 81
  close-grip bench press, 78
  Cybex weight-assisted parallel bar
    dips, 77
  incline dumbbell curl, 72
  low pulley curl, 73
  lying triceps extension, 78
  Nautilus arm curl, 71
  Nautilus triceps extension, 75
  parallel bar dips, 76
  reverse curl, 72
  reverse wrist curl, 81
  seated dumbbell curl, 75
  standing triceps extension, 74
  Universal arm curl, 71
  Universal dip, 79
  Universal triceps extension, 77
Athletes, 1–2, 17
Athletic performance, 2, 10
Atrophy, 7

Back exercises
  back extension, 106
  barbell rowing, 52
  bent-arm pullover, 48
  chin-ups, 54
  Cybex back extension, 107
  Cybex seated rowing, 53
  Cybex weight-assisted pull-up, 55
  low pulley shoulder shrug, 57
  Nautilus seated rowing, 53
  Nautilus pullover, 49
  Nautilus shoulder shrug, 579

one-dumbbell rowing, 57
pull-ups, 54
pull-ups behind the neck, 56
seated low pulley cable rowing, 57
shoulder shrug, 56
Universal bent-arm pullover, 49
Universal lat pulldown, 55
Universal seated back extension,
  107
Back extension, 106
  Cybex machine, 107
  trunk extension, 106, 107
Ball-and-socket joint, 12
Barbell curl, 13, 14, 70
Barbell rowing, 52
Barbell wrist curl, 80
Basic lifts
  cleans, 32
  dead lift, 1, 31, 85
Bench dips, 76
Bench press, 1, 17, 34, 42
Bench step, 88
Bent-arm flyes, 46
Bent-arm pullover
  chest/back exercise, 48
  Nautilus machine, 49
  Universal machine, 49
Bent-over lateral raise, 67
Biceps, 54, 56, 71, 72, 73
Biceps brachii, 54, 56, 70–73
Body builders, 1, 9, 17, 39, 114
Body fat, 8, 9
Body Master
  leg curl, 93
  leg extension, 92
  triceps extension,
Body position, 24
Boss dip machine, 77
Brachialis, 70, 71, 72, 73
Brachioradialis, 70, 71, 72, 73
Breathing, 23–24, 28, 33

Calcium, 110
Calf press
  on Body Master Leg Press
    machine, 96
  on Cybex leg press, 97
Calf raise
  Cybex standing, 95
  one-dumbbell, 96, 162
  seated, 97
  standing, 94
Carbohydrates, 112, 114
Cardiovascular endurance, 9
Central nervous system, 14
Cheating, 154
Chest exercises
  bench press, 1, 17, 34, 42
  bent-arm flyes, 46
  bent-arm pullover, 48
  Boss incline bench press, 45
  Cybex incline bench press, 45
  Cybex seated chest press, 43
  incline bench press, 44–45
  incline dumbbell bench press, 44
  Nautilus 10-degree chest, 47
  Nautilus pullover, 49
  Universal bent-arm pullover, 49

Universal chest press, 47
Universal pec deck, 47
Universal prone bench press, 43
Chest press
  Universal machine, 47
Chin-ups, 54
Cholesterol, 114
Cleans, 32
Clean-and-jerk lift, 1
Close-grip bench press, 78
  Smith machine, 79
Clothing, 21–22
Communication, 26
Concentration, 24, 34
Concentric contraction, 14, 23, 39
Concentric failure, 153
Contractility, 11
Contraction, 8, 11–14, 22–23
Coordination, 9
Coracobrachialis, 66
Crunches, 100, 104, 162
Curl-ups, 100, 162
Cybex Machine exercises
  abdominal machine, 101
  back extension, 107
  hip extension, 90
  hip flexion, 91
  leg press, 89
  seated chest press, 43
  seated lateral raise, 67
  seated overhead press, 63
  seated rowing, 53
  standing calf raise, 95
  weight-assisted parallel bar dips,
    77
  weight-assisted pull-up, 55
Cybex 350 Extremity Testing and
  Rehabilitation System, 14
Cycling, 155

Dead lift, 1, 31, 84, 85
Definition, 1
Dehydration, 109
DeLorme, Dr. Thomas, 156
Deltoid, 60–68
Diet, 114
Dip
  Boss machine, 77
Drugs, 118–120
Dumbbell bench press, 42, 161
Dumbbell squat, 84
Dumbbells, 18, 28, 29–30

Eccentric contraction, 14, 23
Eccentric failure, 154
Elasticity, 11
Emotional development, 5
Endomysium, 12
Endurance, 144, 146
Epimysium, 12
Equipment
  Constant external resistance, 156
  Isokinetic, 156
  Variable resistance, 156
Erector spinae, 31–32, 84, 85, 86,
  106, 107
Evaluating progress, 129–130
Excitability, 11

Exercise form, 22–23, 28, 29–31, 34
Extension, 8, 12, 17, 22
Extensibility, 11

Fats, 112–113
Fat tissue, 7
Finger flexors, 85
Fixed load, 145
Flexibility, 8, 9, 17–18, 23, 25
Flexion, 12
Food Guide Pyramid, (U.S. Dept. of
  Agriculture's), 114–116
Food supplements, 116
Forced reps, 153
Free weights, 29, 33
Frequency, 33, 145
Front raise, 66

Gastrocnemius, 94, 96, 97
Genetic potential, 129
Gluteus maximus, 31–32, 84–91
Goals, 139–141, 143
Grips
  mixed, 29–30
  pronated, 29, 32
  supinated, 30

Hack Squat, 89
Hammer strength arm curl, 73
Hamstrings, 84–86, 90, 93
Hand flexors, 72, 80
Hanging knee raises, 105
Hanging reverse crunches, 105
Heel raise
  Universal machine, 95
Hernia, 9
Hip extension
  Cybex hip extension, 90
  Cybex hip flexion, 91
  dead lift, 1, 31, 85
  dumbbell squat, 84
  leg press, 89
  lunge, 88
  Nautilus leg press, 87
  squat, 84
  step-up, 88
  Universal leg press, 87
  Universal squat, 86
Hip flexion
  Cybex machine, 90
  sit-ups, 102
Home training program, 159
Hormones, 7, 118
Hyperextension, 17

Iliopsoas, 91, 102, 104–105
Incline bench press, 44–45
  Boss, 45
  Cybex, 45
Incline dumbbell bench press, 44
Incline dumbbell curl, 72
Injuries, 9
Intensity, 24
Isokenetic contraction, 14
Isometric contraction, 13
Isotonic contraction, 13–14

Joint capsule, 19
Joint stability, 18

Knee extensions
  Body Master leg curl, 93
  Body Master leg extension, 92
  Nautilus leg extension, 92
  Nautilus seated leg curl, 93
  Universal leg extension, 92
Knee flexion, 93
Knee raises, 105

Lat pulldown
  Universal machine, 55
Lateral raise, 64, 161
  Cybex machine, 66
  dumbbell, 65
Latissimus dorsi, 48–49, 52–55
Lean body mass, 118
Leg curl
  Universal machine, 95
  Nautilus seated, 93
Leg exercises
  barbell squat, 84
  calf press on Body Master Leg
    Press machine, 96
  calf press on Cybex leg press, 97
  Cybex hip extension, 90
  Cybex hip flexion, 91
  Cybex leg press, 86
  dead lift, 1, 31, 84, 85
  dumbbell squat, 84
  lunge, 88
  Nautilus leg press, 87
  one-dumbbell calf raise, 96
  seated calf raise, 97
  squat, 84
  standing barbell calf raise, 94
  standing calf raise, Cybex
    machine, 95
  step up, 88
  Universal heel raise, 95
  Universal leg press, 87
Leg press, 89
  Cybex machine, 86
  Nautilus machine, 87
  Universal machine, 87
Levator scapulae, 56, 57
Ligaments, 18, 19, 25
Low pulley curl, 73
Low pulley shoulder shrug, 57
Low pulley upright rowing
  Universal machine, 63
Lunge, 88, 162
Lying barbell triceps extension, 78

Machines, 24–26, 33, 34
  safety, 28–29
Macronutrients, 109
Measurements
  body fat, 129
  body weight, 129
  muscular endurance, 127
  size, 127–129
  strength, 127
Medical clearance, 21
Mental development, 5
Mental preparation, 17
Mesomorphs, 117
Metabolic rate, 7
Micronutrients, 109
Military press, 60
Minerals, 109–110
Mixed grip, 30–31
Motivation, 157
Muscle size, 144
Muscle tissue, 7
Muscular endurance, 10
Muscular system, 4, 11
Muscle atrophy, 15
Muscle hypertrophy, 15

Muscle fibers, 12
Muscle fitness, 145–146
Muscle tissue
  cardiac, 11
  smooth, 11
  skeletal, 11
Muscle tone, 145–146
Myofibrils, 12
Myofilaments, 12
Myosin, 13

National Academy of Sciences, 109
National Strength and Conditioning
    Association, 3
Nautilus machine exercises
  abdominal crunch, 101
  arm curl, 71
  leg press, 87
  pullover, 49
  seated leg curl, 935
  seated rowing, 53
  shoulder shrug, 57
  10-degree chest, 47
  triceps extension, 75
Negatives, 154
Nutrition, 7, 34, 109–116

Olympic Games, 8
Olympic lifters, 1, 9, 17
One dumbbell calf raise, 96, 162
One-dumbbell rowing, 52, 161
1-Repetition maximum, (1-RM), 3
Overhead lifts, 3
Overhead press
  Boss machine, 61
Overload, 117, 143
Overtraining, 33, 153

Parallel bar dips, 78
Partner, training, 26
Patients, 2
Pectoralis major, 42–49, 668, 76–79
Perimysium, 12
Periodization, 154
Physical fitness, 2, 9–10
Physical preparation, 17
Positive thinking, 1382
Posterior deltoid, 52–53
Power lifters, 1, 9, 17
Progression, 143, 145, 149
Progressive overload, 153
Progressive resistance, 1, 2
Pronated grip, 29, 32
Prone bench press
  Universal machine, 43
Proteins, 113–114
Pullover
  Nautilus machine, 49
Pull-ups, 54

Quadriceps, 31–32, 84–89, 92

Range of motion, 18, 22–23, 25
Record keeping, 125–126
Recruitment, 15
Rectus abdominis, 100–105
Rectus femoris, 91, 102
Rehabilitation, 2
Repetitions, 34, 127, 144, 146
Resistance, 33–34, 144
Rest, 7, 34, 117–118, 144
Results, 138
Reverse crunches, 103
  seated, 104
  hanging, 105
Reverse curl, 72
Reverse wrist curl, 81
Rhomboids, 31, 52–53, 67, 85

Safety, 28, 30
Sarcomere, 12

Seat belts, 24
Seated back extension
  Universal machine, 107
Seated calf raise, 97
Seated chest press
  Cybex machine, 43
Seated dumbbell curl, 70, 161
Seated lateral raise
  Cybex machine, 65
Seated leg curl
  Nautilus machine, 93
Seated reverse crunches, 104
Seated rowing
  Cybex machine, 53
  Nautilus machine, 53
Sedentary lifestyle, 3
Sets, 144
Shoulder exercises
  Boss overhead press machine, 61
  bent-over lateral raise, 67
  Cybex seated lateral raise, 65
  Hammer strength overhead press,
    61
  front raise, 66
  lateral raise, 64
  military press, 60
  Universal low pulley upright row-
    ing, 63
  upright rowing, 62
Shoulder shrug
  upper back (traps), 56
  Nautilus machine, 57
Sit-ups, 102
Size, 146
Skeletal muscles, 11
Snatch lift, 1
Social development, 5–6
Soleus, 94, 96, 97
Specificity, 143
Speed, 25
Spiritual development, 6
Split routine, 154
Spot reduction, 8
Spotting techniques, 3
Squat
  barbell, 84
  barbell squat in power rack, 85
  dumbbell, 89
  front, 90
  hack, 89
  hip and knee extension, 86
  Universal machine, 86
Squat lift, 1
Standing barbell calf raise, 94
Standing calf raise, 97
Standing triceps extension, 76
Static stretching, 19
Step up, 88
Steroids, 118–119
Straight-arm pullover
  dumbbell, 48
Strength, 144, 146
Stretching, 17–20
Supinated grip, 30, 32
Symmetry, 1
Systems
  aerobic circuit, 155
  circuit, 155
  cycling, 155
  double progressive, 154
  giant sets, 155
  one set to failure, 155
  set, 155
  rest-pause, 155
  simple progressive, 154
  super set, 155

10-degree chest
  Nautilus, 47
Tendons, 12, 18–19, 25
Teres major, 52–55

Testosterone, 2, 8, 15, 114
Tobacco, 118–119, 120
Total body routines, 158
Trapezius, 31–32, 52–53, 56, 57,
    62, 63, 64, 65, 67, 85
Triceps extension
  barbell, 74
  Body Master, 79
  lying barbell, 78
  one-dumbbell, 74, 162
  Nautilus machine, 77
  Universal machine, 77
Triceps, 42–45, 62–63, 65, 74–79
Trunk extension
  back extension, 106
  Cybex back extension, 107
  Universal seated back extension,
    107
Trunk Flexion
  crunches, 100
  curl-ups, 100
  hanging knee raises, 105
  Nautilus abdominal crunch
    machine, 101
  reverse crunches, 103
  seated reverse crunches, 104
  sit-ups, 102
  tuck-ups, 103
Tuck-ups, 103

Universal Machine exercises
  arm curl, 71
  bent-arm pullover, 49
  chest press, 47
  dip, 77
  heel raise, 95
  lat pulldown, 55
  leg curl, 93
  leg extension, 92
  leg press, 87
  low pulley upright rowing, 63
  pec deck, 47
  prone bench press, 43
  seated back extension, 107
  squat, 86
  triceps pushdown, 75
Upper back (traps) exercises
  low pulley shoulder shrug, 57
  Nautilus shoulder shrug, 57
  shoulder shrug, 56
Upright rowing, 64
U.S. Department of Health and
    Human Services, 112

Variable load, 145
Variable method, 145
Variable systems
  continuous, 156
  DeLorme, 156
  light to heavy, 156
  percentage, 155
  pyramid, 155
  tonnage, 156
Vitamins, 110–112
Voluntary muscle, 11

Warm-up, 17
Water, 109, 112
Weight-assisted parallel bar dips
  Cybex machine, 77
Weight-assisted pull-up
  Cybex machine, 55
Weight gain, 116
Weight loss, 116
Weight trainers, 2
Work-rest principle, 144
Wrist Curl
  Barbell, 80
  Dumbbell, 80
Wrist flexors, 72, 80
Wrist extensors, 81